OSCEsmart

50 medical student OSCEs
in Surgery

Dr. Nabeel Merali

Executive Consulting Editor:
Dr. Sam Thenabadu

Ordering Information: Quantity sales. Special discounts are available on quantity purchases by corporations, associations, and others. For details, contact the publisher at the address above.

Orders by UK trade bookstores and wholesalers please visit www.scowenpublishing.com

Although every effort has been made to check this text, it is possible that errors have been made, readers are urged to check with the most up to date guidelines and safety regulations.

Publisher's Cataloging-in-Publication data : OSCEsmart 50 medical student OSCEs in Surgery

Copyright © 2017 Simon Cowen Publishing

ISBN: 0-9908538-5-3
ISBN-13: 978-0-9908538-5-5

DEDICATION

' With thanks to my dear parents, my beautiful wife for their support and to Dr. Sam Thenabadu a truly great inspiration and dear friend.'
Nabeel

'For Ammi, Molly, Reuben and Rafa - I.L.Y.T.T.M.'
Sam

CONTENTS

The Acute Abdomen (AAA)

The Acute Abdomen (Pancreatitis)

Right Iliac Fossa Pain in a Female

Bowel Obstruction

Change in Bowel Habits

Anorectal Pain

Bleeding per rectum

Upper Gastrointestinal Bleeding

Obstructive Jaundice

GORD, Dyspepsia, Dysphagia

Right upper quadrant abdominal pain

Peripheral Vascular Disease

Haematuria

Testicular Swelling

Loin to Groin Pain

Neck Swelling

Breast Lump
Pre-Operative Assessment of the High Risk Surgical patient

Blood Transfusion
Conversation on DNAR
Post-operative confusion
Consent for Flexible Sigmoidoscopy
Breaking Bad News

Anxious Relative
Patient wants to Self-discharge
PCA explanation
Epidural analgesia explanation
Referring a patient ITU
Escalation of a sick patient

Suturing under local anaesthetic
Scrubbing
ATLS – C- Spine Immobilization and Rigid Collar
Management of airway including adjuncts
Surgical Chest Drain insertion
Femoral arterial blood Sampling
Ankle Brachial Pressure Index
Male catheterisation
Female Catheterisation
Insertion of a Nasogastric Tube
Abdominal Radiograph Interpretation
Chest Radiograph Interpretation

Examination of an Abdominal Stoma
Examination of an Acute Abdomen
Digital Rectal Examination
Examination of Hernial Orifices
Breast Examination
Neck Lump and Thyroid examination
Examination of Male Genitalia
ATLS Primary Survey
Peripheral Vascular Disease Examination

Introduction to OSCESmart

Doctors of all seniorities can remember the stress of the OSCE but even more so the stress of trying to study and practice for the OSCEs. A multitude of generic undergraduate and postgraduate resources can be found on line but quality, quantity, and completeness of content can vary. The aim of the OSCESmart editorial team is to bring together specialty focused books that have identified 50 core stations encompassing the essential categories of history taking, examinations, emergency moulages, clinical skills and data interpretation with a strong theme of communications running through all the stations.

The combined experience of consultants, registrars and junior doctors to write, edit and quality check these stations, promises to deliver content that is appropriate to reach a standard we would expect of new junior doctors entering their foundation internship years and into core training. It is important to know that these stations are all newly written and based at the level of clinical competencies we would expect from these grades of doctors. Learning objectives exist for undergraduate curricula and for the foundation years, and the scenarios are based and written around these. What they are not, are scenarios that have been 'borrowed' from any medical school.

Preparation is the key to success in most things, but never more so than for the OSCEs and a candidate that hasn't practised will soon be found out. These books will allow you to practice relevant scenarios with verified checklists to learn both content and the generic approach. The format will allow you to practice in groups with one person being the candidate, one the actor and one the examiner. Each scenario finishes with three learning points. Picture these as are three core learning tips that we would want you to take away if you had only a couple of days left to the exam. These OSCE scenarios promise to be a robust revision aide for the student looking to recap and consolidate for their exams, but equally importantly prepare them for life in clinical practice.

I am immensely proud of this OSCESmart series. I have had the pleasure of working with some of the brightest and most dynamic young clinicians and educators I know, and I am sure you will find this series covering the essential clinical specialties a truly robust and invaluable companion in those stressful times of revision. I must take this opportunity to thank my colleagues for all their hard work but most of all to thank my wonderful wife Molly for her unerring love and support and my sons Reuben and Rafael for all the joy they bring me.

Despite the challenging times the health service finds itself in, being a doctor remains a huge privilege. We hope that this OSCESmart series goes some way to help you achieve the excellence you and your patients deserve.
Best of luck, Dr Sam Thenabadu, 2016

Introduction to OSCESmart 50 OSCES in Surgery:

Written by junior doctors, for the junior doctors of tomorrow. This book takes a fresh approach to passing surgical OSCE exams by emphasising on the importance of practicing clinical vignettes with fellow candidates as a team and experiencing the virtue of OSCE role-play.

This book is designed to cover a broad base of core knowledge and skills that will be useful not only in your exam preparation for medical school and MRCS, but also throughout your Doctor Life.

We present a range of fifty scenarios divided into four main chapters, demonstrating the breadth and variety of clinical experience you could expect from a career in the world of surgery. Focused history taking on common surgical topics, difficult communication scenarios, clear clinical topics and surgical examinations are covered in depth by authors who have been through the process.

Our book has clear, step-by-step guides to each clinical station followed by key tips to remember just before you sit the exam, providing a concrete base for students to excel upon. The theme of clear communication runs throughout the book, reflecting its central importance to good clinical care. As well as useful data analyses on how to systematically describe an abdominal radiograph with signs coupled with MRCS syllabus scenarios and examinations.

I can guarantee that using our surgical OSCE revision book coupled with the OSCE Smart series will ease your exam preparation and tee you up for future success.

I would like to thank my co-authors, for their wonderful dedication, collaborative spirit and priceless work. As well as to Sam Thenabadu for all your wise words of wisdom, teaching and inspiration.

Nabeel

About the authors

Dr Nabeel Merali

Nabeel Merali qualified from Barts & London Medical School in 2012 and undertook his foundation training in South Thames London deanery. Having attained a Merit award in Laparoscopic Surgical Skills & Science Masters in 2015 at Barts Cancer Institute with a keen interest in laparoscopic simulation training for students.

He is currently a general themed core surgical trainee at Frimley Park Hospital, Kent, Surrey and Sussex (KSS) Deanery. He has a strong interest in teaching, designing local medical student OSCE sessions and keeping fit by playing football.

Dr Sam Thenabadu
MBBS MRCP DRCOG DCH MA Clin Ed FRCEM MSc (Paed) FHEA

Consultant Adult & Paediatric Emergency Medicine
Honorary Senior Lecturer & Associate Director of Medical Education

Sam Thenabadu graduated from King's College Medical School in 2001 and dual trained in Adult and Paediatric Emergency Medicine in London before being appointed a consultant in 2011 at the Princess Royal University Hospital. He has Masters degrees in Clinical Medical Education and Advanced Paediatrics.

He is undergraduate director of medical education at the King's College NHS Trust and the academic block lead for Emergency Medicine and Critical Care at King's College School of Medicine. At postgraduate level he has been the Pan London Health Education England lead for CT3 paediatric emergency medicine trainees since 2011. Academically he has previously written two textbooks and has published in peer review journals and given numerous oral and poster presentations at national conferences in emergency medicine, paediatrics, medical education and patient quality and safety.

He has an unashamed passion for medical education and strives to achieve excellence for himself, his colleagues and his patients, hoping to always deliver this through an enjoyable learning environment. Service delivery and educational need not be two separate entities, and he hopes that those who have had great teachers will take it upon themselves to do the same for others in the future.

Co-Authors

Dr. Debo Adebayo BMBS, MClinEd,
Foundation Year 2, London

Dr. Adam Garland MBBS, BSc,
Foundation Year 2, London

Dr. Frederick Hartley, MBBS, MRCS,
Core Surgical Trainee Year 2, London

Major Max Marsden MBBS BSc DMCC DOHNS MRCS,
Clinical Research Fellow, General Surgery Registrar, Military Deanery

Dr Sarah Schneider, MBChB, BMedSci Hons,
Emergency Medicine trainee (ACCS) CT1, London

Dr Daniel Thompson MBBS, BAHons,
Anatomy Demonstrator King's College London

Dr. Thomas Thompson, MBBS, BSc,
Foundation Year 2, London

Abbreviations

AAA – Abdominal aorta aneurysm
ABCDE – Airway, Breathing, Circulation, Disability, Exposure
ATLS – Advance Trauma Life Support
BD – Twice a day
BPH - Benign Prostatic Hyperplasia
BPM – Beats Per Minute
C-Spine – Cervical Spine
CT - Computerised tomography
CT IVU - Computerised tomography intravenous urogram
CXR – Chest Radiograph
DNAR - Do Not Attempt Resuscitation
DRE – Digital Rectal Examination
ERCP - Endoscopic Retrograde cholangiopancreatography
FNA- Fine Needle Aspiration
GORD - Gastro-oesophageal reflux disease
GP - General practitioner
ITU – Intensive Care Unit
IHD – Ischemic Heart Disease
MRCP - Magnetic resonance cholangiopancreatography
RUQ- Right upper quadrant
OD – Once a day
OSCEs - objective structured clinical examinations
PCA – Pain Control Analgesia
PRN- As when Required
PSA – Prostate-specific antigen
P-POSSUM – risk calculation in a preoperative patient
SOCRATES - mnemonic acronym used evaluate the nature of pain
TIA- Transient Ischemic Attack
USS - Ultrasound

Chapter One

History Taking Scenarios

1. Acute Abdomen (AAA)

Student vignette

A 72-year-old man has presented to the Emergency department acutely unwell with severe abdominal pain.

You are the foundation year doctor on the surgical team and have been asked to take the initial history and then summarise your findings back to the surgical registrar on-call.

After 6 minutes the examiner will stop you and ask you to summarise back your findings, suggest your differential diagnoses and your initial management plan.

Actor Instructions:

You are a 72-year-old man named Charles, who is attending Emergency department due to the sudden onset of a severe pain in your abdomen. You have had some grumbling type pains for several months and thought it was indigestion.

This afternoon when you were reading the paper when a sudden pain started in the centre of your abdomen that made you double over, feel very faint and almost lose consciousness. It is a very sharp pain and at its worst is 9/10 in severity. The pain is also felt in your back. The paracetamol that you had when it came on has not touched it and you are beginning to feel hot and sweaty as well as very nauseous. Nothing appears to be making it better or worse and you are feeling increasingly anxious about what it might be. You have been opening your bowels normally and have not lost any weight recently.

Generally you are quite fit and well and are a retired Civil Servant who still finds time to play regular golf. You live at home with your partner and travel extensively. You remember your GP years ago putting you on a medication for high blood pressure but you stopped taking it because you didn't like the taste and have never been back. You are not currently taking any regular medications and have only had one operation in the past where they removed your gallbladder. You are an only child and remember that your father had a sudden death when you were young but that your mother never explained why.

You are intermittently very distressed because of the pain. Try to get the doctor to tell you what he thinks is going on and question whether you are going to die?

Examiner Instructions:

A 72-year-old man has presented to the Emergency department acutely unwell with severe abdominal pain. The foundation year doctor has been asked to take the initial history and summarise their findings.

After 6 minutes stop the candidate and ask them to 'please summarise your findings, including a differential diagnosis and immediate management plan' for 2 minutes.

Please follow the mark sheet and grade appropriately.

Marksheet: Acute Abdomen (Aortic Aneurysm)

Task	Achieved	Not Achieved
Wash hands & Introduces self		
Clarifies who they are speaking to		
Elicits presenting complaint		
Offers reassurance and calms patient		
History of presenting complaint		
Explores differentials – asks about pain (SOCRATES)		
Explores associated symptoms		
Asks about whether the symptoms fluctuate		
Explores differentials – asks about red flags of malignancy		
Asks about past medical & surgical history		
Asks about Drug History, allergies		
Ask about Family History & Social History		
Summarises history concisely		
Explains further immediate management (Approach using an ABCDE technique)		
Leaking AAA top of differentials, name three more		
Mentions this is an emergency & resuscitation		
Mention the need for close monitoring, Access, Blood markers, G&S clotting and order units of RBC		
Escalate to your senior		
Notify Emergency theatres and anaesthetist on call		
If patient is clinically stable, discuss forms of imaging such as CT angiogram		
Examiner's Global Mark	/5	
Actor/Helper Global Mark	/5	
Total	/30	

4

Learning Points:

Learn by heart the differential diagnoses of the acute abdomen presentation. SOCRATES is a mnemonic acronym for pain assessment, Site/Onset/Character/ Radiation/ Associations/ Time course/ Exacerbating/relieving factors/ Severity of pain score. Remember this tool for every history taking

Make sure your History taking includes important negatives to help you work towards your top diagnosis.

Always immediately manage acutely unwell patients using the **A B C D E** approach.

2. Acute Abdomen (Pancreatitis)

Student vignette

A 31-year-old male has been brought into Emergency Department by ambulance with severe abdominal pain.

You are the foundation year doctor on the surgical team and have been asked to take the initial history and then summarise your findings back to the surgical registrar on-call.

After 6 minutes the examiner will stop you and ask you to summarise back your findings, suggest your differential diagnoses and your initial management plan.

Actor Instructions:

You are a 31-year-old male named Christopher, who has just got off a particularly heavy weekend of drinking. Today you were suddenly overcome by a sharp, pain in your central abdomen. The pain is currently 10/10 in severity and extremely debilitating. It feels as if it is burning a hole into your back and you have vomited on multiple occasions with it. Painkillers have not helped, but sitting still is the only thing that sometimes helps it.

Otherwise you had been generally well up until today.

You were out partying this weekend and consumed approximately 12 pints of normal strength lager and half a bottle of vodka.

If questioned you will admit to drinking a bit more than you used and average around 10 units per day, often needing a drink before midday.

You have noticed a reduction in your appetite recently. You have never been to Hospital before for anything.

You have had no recent foreign travel, take the odd line of cocaine but no injectable drugs and smoke 10 cigarettes per day. Your father was a big drinker too but you don't know of any other family conditions. You have no allergies and do not take any medication regularly except for ibuprofen from time to time when you get muscle aches.

You are very agitated throughout the consultation and should demand pain relief several times. If the doctor appears empathic and explains that he needs to find out what is wrong to best help you then you relent somewhat.

Examiner Instructions:

A 31-year-old male has been brought into Emergency Department by ambulance with severe abdominal pain. The foundation year doctor has been asked to take the initial history and summarise their findings.

After 6 minutes stop the candidate and ask them to 'please summarise your findings, including a differential diagnosis and immediate management plan' for 2 minutes.

Please follow the mark sheet and grade appropriately.

Marksheet: Acute Abdomen (Pancreatitis)

Task	Achieved	Not Achieved
Wash hands & Introduces self		
Clarifies who they are speaking to		
Elicits presenting complaint		
Offers reassurance and calms patient		
History of presenting complaint		
Explores differentials – asks about pain (SOCRATES)		
Explores associated symptoms		
Asks about whether the symptoms fluctuate		
Explores differentials – asks about red flags of malignancy		
Asks about past medical & surgical history		
Asks about Drug History, allergies		
Ask about Family History & Social History		
Asks patient about their alcohol intake		
Specifically gets the patient to quantify their recent alcohol intake		
Elicits at least one concerning factor related to alcoholism (unemployed, eye opener, lack of appetite, family history)		
Summarises history concisely		
Explains further immediate management (Approach using an ABCDE technique)		
Perforated peptic ulcer or pancreatitis as top of differentials, name three more		
Escalate to your senior, ABG, Erect CXR, blood profile including amylase		
Examiner's Global Mark	/5	
Actor/Helper Global Mark	/5	
Total	/30	

Learning Points:

Know the mnemonic for causes of Pancreatitis: I GET SMASHED.

Pancreatitis patients can be critically unwell – be familiar with the Glasgow Score as a means of assessing this.

Use the CAGE questionnaire for a quick assessment of alcohol dependence (Thought of Cutting down/Anger at people criticizing your drinking/Guilt about your drinking/Eye-opener the morning after).

3.Right Iliac Fossa Pain in a Female

Student vignette

A 22-year-old female has been brought into Emergency Department by ambulance with right iliac fossa pain for the last 12 hours.

You are the foundation year doctor on the surgical team and have been asked to take the initial history and then summarise your findings back to the surgical registrar on-call.

After 6 minutes the examiner will stop you and ask you to summarise back your findings, suggest your differential diagnoses and your initial management plan.

Actor Instructions:

You are a 22-year-old history student named Lisa. For the last 12 hours you've been experiencing severe abdominal pain. The pain woke you up from your sleep. The pain started in the right iliac fossa and you can feel it below your belly button too. The pain is quite sharp; it's 7 out of 10 and seems to come in waves but never totally goes away.

The pain started very suddenly. You took some paracetamol earlier and that seems to have helped with the pain a bit. Lying still makes the pain feel a bit better as well. Walking makes it worse. The pain is making you feel sick and you've lost your appetite. You have not vomited. You had one loose bowel motion this morning.

You have some mild increase in urinary frequency but no dysuria. You've passed urine 5 times in the last few hours. Your boyfriend drove you to hospital and the car journey felt uncomfortable. You don't feel feverish; you've got no joint pain or muscle soreness. No one else at home is unwell. You've not travelled abroad recently or eating from takeaways.

You've recently had a sexual transmitted disease check-up, which was negative. You have one male sexual partner. You have no vaginal discharge. You are not currently using contraception. You're mid-cycle and normally have a regular 28-day cycle. You don't think you're pregnant.

You had a laparoscopy under the gynecologists last year for a similar pain and were told you had endometriosis. You haven't had any other operations. You suffer with hay fever and take an antihistamine in the summer but you can't remember the name. You have asthma and use a blue inhaler. You don't have any drug allergies.

You're a non-smoker drink alcohol socially and don't use illicit drugs. You live with your boyfriend You have no relevant family history and no other symptoms.

Examiner Instructions:

A 22-year-old female has been brought into Emergency Department by ambulance with right iliac fossa pain for the last 12 hours. The foundation year doctor has been asked to take the initial history and summarise their findings.

After 6 minutes stop the candidate and ask them to 'please summarise your findings, including a differential diagnosis and immediate management plan' for 2 minutes.

Please follow the mark sheet and grade appropriately.

Marksheet: Right Iliac Fossa Pain in a Female

Task	Achieved	Not Achieved
Wash hands & Introduces self		
Clarifies who they are speaking to		
Elicits presenting complaint		
Offers reassurance and calms patient		
History of presenting complaint		
Explores differentials – asks about pain (SOCRATES)		
Asks about exacerbating/relieving factors		
Asks about urinary symptoms		
Asks about sexual history		
Asks about menstrual history		
Asks about past medical & surgical history		
Asks about Drug History, allergies		
Ask about Family History & Social History		
Explore Ideas, Concerns, Expectations		
Summarises history concisely		
Presents a reasonable differential diagnosis (3 of ectopic pregnancy, appendicitis, ovarian pathology, urinary tract infection)		
Next management steps to include examination of the patient's abdomen		
Specifically mentions the need for urine dip test and pregnancy test		
Specifically mentions the importance of inflammatory marker blood tests		
Discuss imaging, organising ultrasound abdomen/pelvis		
Examiner's Global Mark	/5	
Actor/Helper Global Mark	/5	
Total	/30	

Learning Points:

Appendicitis is the most common surgical emergency but in women of childbearing age ectopic pregnancy must always be considered. A joint care approach with Gynaecology may be needed in the first instance as delay must never occur with disagreements around which team should be in charge.

For women with normal inflammatory markers and sudden onset right iliac fossa pains consider gynaecological causes.

The Alvarado score has a low sensitivity but remembering the points of the score helps to collect many of the clinically relevant pieces of information.

4. Bowel Obstruction

Student vignette

A 70-year-old man has been referred directly to the on-call surgical registrar by his GP with abdominal pain and vomiting.

You are the foundation year doctor on the surgical team and have been asked to take the initial history and then summarise your findings back to the surgical registrar on-call.

After 6 minutes the examiner will stop you and ask you to summarise back your findings, suggest your differential diagnoses and your initial management plan.

Actor Instructions:

You are a 70-year-old man named Alex, you made an appointment with your GP today because of 2 days of worsening central abdominal pain and 24 hours of persistent vomiting.

The pain is much worse on movement and you are most comfortable laying flat. It is a moderately severe constant pain. You were mostly concerned by the fact that you have been vomiting everything you try to swallow. The rest of the time you are vomiting bile and have not been able to take your regular medications. You feel that this is just a stomach bug and don't understand why the GP sent you to hospital, you only wanted a medicine for the vomiting.

You had also developed an increased frequency in opening your bowels in those 3 months. You last opened your bowels 4 days ago. When probed you realize that you have not passed wind for at least a day, maybe more.

You suffer from high blood pressure, diabetes and atrial fibrillation. You had polyps removed from the bowel 4 years ago. You are on many medications but cannot remember their names. You are not aware of any specific illnesses in the family.

You have smoked 10 cigarettes a day for at least 50 years. You don't drink alcohol and used to work as a HGV driver. You admit to have been very unhealthy in your working years.

If asked you have noticed reduced appetite for a while and have gone down at least 3 notches on your belt in the past 3 months.

If asked about other symptoms: you have noticed only- pallor of the face, shortness of breath on walking and increased lethargy.

Examiner Instructions:

A 70-year-old man has been referred directly to the on-call surgical registrar by his GP with abdominal pain and vomiting. The foundation year doctor has been asked to take the initial history and summarise their findings.

After 6 minutes stop the candidate and ask them to 'please summarise your findings, including a differential diagnosis and immediate management plan' for 2 minutes.

Please follow the mark sheet and grade appropriately.

Marksheet: Right Iliac Fossa Pain in a Female

Task	Achieved	Not Achieved
Wash hands & Introduces self		
Clarifies who they are speaking to		
Elicits presenting complaint		
Offers reassurance and calms patient		
History of presenting complaint		
Explores differentials – asks about pain (SOCRATES)		
Explores associated symptoms		
Explores a full gastro-intestinal history from mouth to anus		
Explores differentials – asks about red flags of malignancy		
Asks about change in bowel habits, absolute constipation, oral intake		
Asks about past medical & surgical history		
Asks about Drug History, allergies		
Ask about Family History & Social History		
Summarises history concisely		
Explores patient's Ideas, Concerns and Expectations		
Addresses patient's belief re diagnosis and desire to leave		
Explains further immediate management (Approach using an ABCDE technique)		
Bowel obstruction top of differentials, name three more		
Mention the need for close monitoring, Access, Blood markers, G&S clotting and order units of RBC		
Recommend NGT, catheter 'drip & suck', IVI, CT abdomen/pelvis		
Examiner's Global Mark	/5	
Actor/Helper Global Mark	/5	
Total	/30	

Learning Points:

Bowel cancer especially caecum pathology is often associated with a new anaemia. Don't forget to ask about anaemia symptoms in your system's enquiry.

Be specific when providing a management plan in an OSCE. Don't just state the test you would order but add why you are doing it and what you are looking for to gain the full marks. Also include name, route and dose of drugs where possible.

Do not neglect the points you will receive for your communication skills. In such a station taking notice of the patient's desire to leave and exploring his Ideas, Concerns and Expectations (ICE) can gain you numerous marks and importantly project a better global impression to the actor and examiner. Ultimately practicing this now will make you a much better doctor too as the success of most consultations rest upon ICE.

5. Change in Bowel Habits

Student vignette

A 62-year-old male has presented to the general surgical clinic with difficulty opening his bowels.

You are the foundation year doctor the surgical team and have been asked to take the initial history and then summarise your findings back to your consultant.

After 6 minutes the examiner will stop you and ask you to summarise back your findings, suggest your differential diagnoses and your initial management plan.

Actor Instructions:

You are a 62-year-old gentleman named Simon, who has been experiencing pain on passing stool for the last week. This pain is mild and is more of a discomfort on defecation. As soon as you pass stool the pain disappeared. You have noticed that your stool has been getting harder. You have been having increasing difficulty-passing stool for the past 2 months, which has been getting worse. You have to strain more and have a feeling that you have not passed everything that is inside.

You have not noticed any bleeding. 10 years ago you had episodes of rectal bleeding and underwent a colonoscopy. This revealed a polyp that was removed.

You have lost 5 kilograms of weight in the last 3 months but should only mention this if asked directly. You did not plan on losing this weight but view it as a good thing as you are overweight.

You also suffer with high blood pressure and take 10mg of amlodipine once a day for this. You do not have any allergies.

Your father developed bowel cancer and had to have part of his bowel removed before he passed away from pneumonia.

You smoke 10 cigarettes a day. You drink alcohol socially. You live with your wife and are fully independent.

You are worried that this could be cancer as your father had it before he died and are scared that you could need an operation.

Examiner Instructions:

A 62-year-old male has presented to the general surgical clinic with difficulty opening his bowels. The foundation year doctor has been asked to take the initial history and summarise their findings.

After 6 minutes stop the candidate and ask them to 'please summarise your findings, including a differential diagnosis and immediate management plan' for 2 minutes.

Please follow the mark sheet and grade appropriately.

Marksheet: Change in bowel habit

Task	Achieved	Not Achieved
Wash hands & Introduces self		
Clarifies who they are speaking to		
Elicits presenting complaint		
Explores patient's pain (SOCRATES)		
Explores associated symptoms		
Elicits timeline of symptoms		
Asks about red flags - Elicits weight loss symptoms		
Asks about red flags – PR bleeding and mucus, tenesmus		
Asks about red flags – appetite		
Asks about red flags – abdominal pain		
Asks about past medical & surgical history		
Asks about Drug History, allergies		
Ask about Family History & Social History		
Asks about past medical & surgical history		
Identifies patient's concerns		
Summarises history concisely		
Explains further immediate management (abdominal and PR examination)		
Provides differential diagnoses (name three)		
Malignancy at top of differentials		
Mentions need for colonoscopy, tumour markers and CT CAP in view of weight loss and staging		
Examiner's Global Mark	/5	
Actor/Helper Global Mark	/5	
Total	/30	

Learning Points:

Colorectal cancer is the 3rd most common malignancy in the UK. Change in bowel habit in the over 50s is bowel cancer until proven otherwise.

Always ask about red flag symptoms. Red flags for colorectal cancer are change in bowel habit, PR bleeding, weight loss, abdominal pain, mucus passed PR and loss of appetite.

Differential diagnoses do exist including diverticulitis, inflammatory bowel disease, irritable bowel disease and local pathologies such as haemorrhoid disease however if red flags exist key investigations for bowel cancer such as colonoscopy with biopsies will be undertaken.

6. Anorectal Pain

Student vignette

A 63-year-old male has presented to hospital with anorectal pain.

You are the foundation year doctor on the general surgical team and have been asked to take the initial history and then summarise your findings back to the registrar on-call.

After 6 minutes the examiner will stop you and ask you to summarise back your findings, suggest your differential diagnoses and your initial management plan.

Actor Instructions:

You are a 53-year-old gentleman called John. You have presented complaining of pain just to the left side of your anus. You are embarrassed about this and are quite reluctant to go into much detail without reassurance. You are afraid that your medical records will have to be sent to your employer and that this embarrassing symptom will be known throughout the office.

This pain started several days ago. It is there constantly and has been getting gradually worse. It is now very painful and tender to touch. You also think that you can feel a swelling that you think is causing the pain. You have tried taking paracetamol, but this has not had much of an effect.

You have also started to feel generally unwell and have been sweating a lot although you feel cold. You have also lost some of your appetite.
You suffer from Type 2 Diabetes Mellitus for which you take insulin and high blood pressure.

Your full medications list is Metformin 1g twice a day, Novomix 30-20 units twice a day, Lisinopril 2.5mg every morning and Simvastatin 40mg at night.
You are allergic to penicillin. You had it as a teenager and it caused your face to swell and made it very hard to breathe.

Your father died of a heart attack aged 72 and your mother is still alive. Nothing runs in the family that you know of.

You smoke 5 cigarettes a day although you are trying to give up. You drink socially. You live with your wife and are fully independent.

Examiner Instructions:

A 53-year-old gentleman has come to the hospital with anorectal pain. The foundation year doctor has been asked to take the initial history and summarise their findings.

After 6 minutes stop the candidate and ask them to 'please summarise your findings, including a differential diagnosis and immediate management plan' for 2 minutes.

Please follow the mark sheet and grade appropriately.

Marksheet:Anorectal Pain

Task	Achieved	Not Achieved
Wash hands & Introduces self		
Clarifies who they are speaking to		
Identifies patient's concerns		
Reassures patient about confidentiality		
Elicits presenting complaint		
Offers reassurance to patient		
Explores patient's pain (SOCRATES)		
Explores associated symptoms		
Elicits timeline of symptoms		
Asks about red flags (bleeding, weight loss, appetite)		
Asks about past medical & surgical history		
Asks about Drug History, allergies		
Ask about Family History & Social History		
Summarises history concisely		
Explains further immediate management (abdominal and PR examination)		
Provides differential diagnoses (name three)		
Perianal Abscess top of differentials		
Mentions this is a surgical emergency		
Offers Incision and Drainage		
Explain the wound will be packed and regularly dressed, healing under secondary intention		
Examiner's Global Mark	/5	
Actor/Helper Global Mark	/5	
Total	/30	

Learning Points:

Some patients will require reassurance regarding confidentiality before they fully divulge information. Everything in this case can stay confidential to yourself and the surgical team. By routinely making this clear at the beginning of consultations, especially those surrounding personal topics, the trust between doctor and patient will be far stronger.

Perianal abscess is a surgical emergency and requires incision and drainage. Therefore know the appropriate next steps. This patient will be needing surgery within 24 hours so will need pre-surgery bloods: FBC, U&E, clotting screen and Group and Save. Analgesia is also paramount with regular medications prescribed and regular review to ensure the pain is being managed.

Remember to think about Inflammatory bowel disease i.e. Crohns in patients who present with perianal abscess and anorectal fistulas. Here surgeons may deal with the initial problem but the abscess may be a harbinger of a more systemic clinical problem that requires joint care with the gastroenterology team.

7. Bleeding per rectum

Student vignette

An 83-year-old male has been brought into Emergency Department by ambulance with abdominal pain and severe rectal bleeding.

You are the foundation year doctor the surgical team and have been asked to take the initial history and then summarise your findings back to the surgical registrar on-call.

After 6 minutes the examiner will stop you and ask you to summarise back your findings, suggest your differential diagnoses and your initial management plan.

Actor Instructions:

You are an 83-Year-old retired soldier named George. Over the last three days you have started to feel generally unwell, tired and grumbling left lower abdominal pain. Tonight you had an intense severe abdominal pain followed by several episodes of bright fresh rectal bleeding. This has never happened before. The pain in the abdomen has stopped, however you continue to have fresh rectal bleeding and are feeling light headed now.

You suffer from high blood pressure, atrial fibrillation and have had a heart attack in 2009. Your full medications list is Lisinopril 2.5mg every morning, Simvastatin 40mg at night, Warfarin once a day, Bisoprolol 2.5mg every morning and GTN spray if required. You have no allergies that you know of.

You live alone, independent and able to walk a few miles without feeling SOB. You occasionally drink a glass of whiskey a night and smoke cigars.

Towards the end of the consultation you start becoming a little concerned that it could be what your father had, which was colon cancer. He wasn't diagnosed until it was too late.

Examiner instructions:

An 83-year-old male has been brought into Emergency Department by ambulance with abdominal pain and severe rectal bleeding. The foundation year doctor has been asked to take the initial history and summarise their findings.

After 6 minutes stop the candidate and ask them to 'please summarise your findings, including a differential diagnosis and immediate management plan' for 2 minutes.

Please follow the mark sheet and grade appropriately.

Marksheet:Bleeding per rectum

Task	Achieved	Not Achieved
Wash hands & Introduces self		
Clarifies who they are speaking to		
Elicits presenting complaint		
Explores patient's pain (SOCRATES)		
Explores associated symptoms		
Elicits timeline of symptoms		
Asks about red flags - Elicits weight loss symptoms		
Asks about red flags – PR bleeding and mucus, tenesmus		
Asks about red flags – appetite		
Asks about red flags – abdominal pain		
Asks about past medical & surgical history		
Asks about Drug History, allergies, Discuss warfarin		
Ask about Family History & Social History		
Asks about past medical & surgical history		
Identifies patient's concerns		
Summarises history concisely		
Explains further immediate management (abdominal and PR examination)		
Provides differential diagnoses (name three)		
Diverticulitis and Malignancy at top of differentials		
ABCDE Resuscitation management, CT Abdomen/Pelvis and management of diverticulitis		
Examiner's Global Mark	/5	
Actor/Helper Global Mark	/5	
Total	/30	

Learning Points:

Always remember to use an ABCDE approach and recognise the common red flag symptoms to look out for in a patient with rectal bleeding. The history should provide clues to narrow down your differential diagnoses.

The most common causes for a severe lower gastrointestinal (GI) bleed is diverticular disease or angiodysplasia. Severe haemorrhage can arise in 3-5% of patients with diverticulosis. The site of bleeding may more often be located in the proximal colon. Presentation is usually abrupt painless bleeding. The patient may have mild lower abdominal cramps or the urge to defecate, followed by passage of a large amount of red or maroon blood or clots. Melaena can occasionally occur but is uncommon.

Conventional colonoscopy is considered the optimal investigation for rectal bleeding. However in some cases a CT triple phase angiogram are requested to pin point the bleeding vessel in emergency situations.

8. Upper Gastrointestinal Bleeding

Student vignette

A 68-year-old female has been brought into Emergency Department by ambulance with haematemesis.

You are the foundation year doctor the surgical team and have been asked to take the initial history and then summarise your findings back to the surgical registrar on-call.

After 6 minutes the examiner will stop you and ask you to summarise back your findings, suggest your differential diagnoses and your initial management plan.

Actor's Instructions:

You are a 68-year-old lady named Jenny, who is panicking after having vomited a large amount of blood this morning. You vomited around 1 pint of blood this morning and immediately called an ambulance. You had a second episode of vomiting in the ambulance bringing up a further half a pint of blood. The blood looks dark red with no clots and nothing mixed in. You have never experienced anything like this before.

You are not in any pain, only scared about the experience and think you are dying. You feel dizzy, especially when you stand up and have stayed on the hospital bed not moving because of this. You have not opened your bowels today. You have not noticed any blood in your stool and it does not look black, although it has looked a bit darker in the last two weeks. You have not passed any urine this morning.

You did not have any episodes of vomiting prior to this. You have not had any reflux or any symptoms of heartburn. You have not had any pain in your abdomen recently. You have not been involved in any trauma. You have no signs of infection and have not been losing any weight.

Only give this information if asked directly. You have been drinking increasing amounts of alcohol ever since your husband passed away of pancreatic cancer one and a half years ago. You drink around 1-2 bottles of wine a night.

You do not have any other medical problems and are not on any regular medications. You have no allergies that you know of.

You live alone since your husband passed away. You have a daughter who moved to Australia 3 months ago. You do not smoke. You drink alcohol as mentioned above.

Examiner's Instructions:

A 68-year-old female has been brought into Emergency Department by ambulance with haematemsis. The foundation year doctor has been asked to take the initial history and summarise their findings.

After 6 minutes stop the candidate and ask them to 'please summarise your findings, including a differential diagnosis and immediate management plan' for 2 minutes.

Please follow the mark sheet and grade appropriately.

Marksheet: Upper GI Bleed

Task	Achieved	Not Achieved
Wash hands & Introduces self		
Clarifies who they are speaking to		
Elicits presenting complaint		
Offers reassurance and calms patient		
History of presenting complaint		
Explores haematemesis – volume, appearance,		
Explores associated symptoms		
Explores differentials – asks about pain		
Explores differentials – asks prior vomiting		
Explores differentials – asks about red flags of malignancy		
Elicits chronic alcohol history		
Elicits reasons for alcoholism		
Asks about past medical & surgical history		
Asks about Drug History, allergies		
Ask about Family History & Social History		
Summarises history concisely		
Explains further immediate management (Approach using an ABCDE technique)		
Variceal Bleeding top of differentials, name three more		
Mentions this is an emergency & resuscitation		
Urgent endoscopy within 4 hours and mention scoring system for UGI Bleeds		
Examiner's Global Mark	/5	
Actor/Helper Global Mark	/5	
Total	/30	

Learning Points:

Oesophageal Variceal bleeding carries a very high mortality rate and requires intravenous terlipressin and urgent endoscopic intervention within 4 hours.

If a patient with haematemesis presented shocked then they will need to be resuscitated and stabilised before endoscopy can occur, remember bleeding severity can be assessed by extent of blood loss and degree of shock. This requires large bore access and fluid resuscitation. Where blood loss is the obvious cause the resuscitation fluid should be blood with O negative blood used if type specific or fully cross matched isnt readily available.

Recommendations emphasise early risk stratification, using the Blatchford score at first assessment and the full Rockall score after endoscopy.

9. Obstructive Jaundice

Student vignette

A 41-year-old lady with right upper quadrant pain is the next patient to be seen on the surgical take list.

You are the foundation year doctor on the surgical team and have been asked to take the initial history and then summarise your findings back to the surgical registrar on-call.

After 6 minutes the examiner will stop you and ask you to summarise back your findings, suggest your differential diagnoses and your initial management plan.

Actor Instructions:

You are a 41-year-old mother of three. You've come to hospital today because you can no longer tolerate the pain in your upper abdomen. The pain is severe, constant, and you can feel it like a band travelling under your right ribs to your back. The pain is worse with eating and hasn't settled since your burger and doughnut last night. You feel nauseated and have vomited several times.

Co-codamol has helped bring the pain down from an 8 to a 6. There are no positions that help you get more comfortable.

You have dark urine and pale stools. You feel feverish and unwell. You had an episode of shaking and shivering last night. You've been feeling hot and cold all day today. No one else at home is unwell. Bowel open normally this morning. No urinary symptoms. Mild headache. You feel very thirsty and extremely itchy.

You had a similar episode 2 years ago, which only lasted 12 hours. Two years ago you went to the GP who gave you omeprazole and organized an USS. He said you had gallstones but nothing needed to be done. Since then you've had intermittent pain which feels like trapped wind normally after eating a big meal but goes away on its own and doesn't last long. This time the pain hasn't gone away. You don't think the omeprazole helps. You've gone yellow and this is new, which is extremely worrying. You've had an appendectomy before. You've been told you're overweight and you developed diabetes in your last two pregnancies.

You only take Omeprazole and are allergic to Penicillin. You're a stay at home mother. You smoke 10 cigarettes a day and don't drink alcohol. You have no other symptoms and no relevant family history. Take all other details from your own experience.

Examiner Instructions:

A 41-year-old lady with right upper quadrant pain is the next patient to be seen on the surgical take list. The foundation year doctor has been asked to take the initial history and summarise their findings.

After 6 minutes stop the candidate and ask them to 'please summarise your findings, including a differential diagnosis and immediate management plan' for 2 minutes.

Please follow the mark sheet and grade appropriately.

Marksheet: Obstructive Jaundice

Task	Achieved	Not Achieved
Wash hands & Introduces self		
Clarifies who they are speaking to		
Elicits presenting complaint		
Offers reassurance and calms patient		
History of presenting complaint		
Explores differentials – asks about pain (SOCRATES)		
Explores associated symptoms		
Pain radiating to the shoulder tip or scapula		
Explores differentials – asks about pain		
Symptoms of obstructive jaundice		
Asks about past medical & surgical history		
Asks about Drug History, allergies		
Ask about Family History & Social History		
Explores patient's Ideas, Concerns and Expectations		
Summarises history concisely		
Explains further immediate management (Approach using an ABCDE technique)		
3 of Acute Cholecystitis, Cholangitis Pancreatitis, Choledocholithiasis, top of differentials, name three more		
Suggests managing the patient immediately using the ABCDE approach		
Specifically mentions 2 of: erect CXR, serum amylase, inflammatory markers or abdominal USS, MRCP (Intraductal stones), ERCP,		
Recommends giving analgesia and antibiotics		
Examiner's Global Mark	/5	
Actor/Helper Global Mark	/5	
Total	/30	

44

Learning Points:

Acute cholecystitis patients can be very unwell with sepsis & jaundice − management of sepsis starts with an A to E assessment and resuscitation following the sepsis 6 care bundle. The main difference from biliary colic and cholecystitis is the inflammatory component (local peritonism, fever, raised white cell count. If the stone moves to the CBD, jaundice may occur.

Use targeted investigations to make a diagnosis following a thorough examination. Ultrasound is the key technique in distinguishing medical from surgical jaundice, and should be performed on all cases of acutely unwell jaundice.

Recommend diagnostic flow chart for patients for intraductal Common bile duct stone is firstly perform MRCP, then ERCP and early laparoscopic cholecystectomy.

10. GORD, Dyspepsia, Dysphagia

Student vignette

A 68-year-old man has been referred to the surgical registrar on call by his GP with severe dysphagia.

You are the foundation year doctor on the surgical team and have been asked to take the initial history and then summarise your findings back to the surgical registrar on-call.

After 6 minutes the examiner will stop you and ask you to summarise back your findings, suggest your differential diagnoses and your initial management plan.

Actor Instructions:

You are a 68-year-old man named Neville, who has been sent to the surgical admission unit by your GP. You made an emergency appointment with your GP earlier today as you have been having difficulty swallowing. You have not been able to swallow any food or liquids other than small sips of water for the past 48hours and feel very unwell. For the past 48hours everything you swallow seems to get stuck and then be regurgitated within a few minutes, undigested. Sometimes this is associated with a sharp pain behind your breastbone.

Thinking back, you believe problems may have started around 6 months ago when you started to have to have softer foods and smaller mouthfuls to be comfortable swallowing your food. In the past month you have been eating soups only. Your wife has been nagging you to see your doctor but you only got concerned these past two days when even water was being regurgitated.
You have lost around 3 stones in weight and have been sleeping a lot more recently.

If asked specifically, you mention that for most of you adult years you had been getting sharp central chest pains. They always seemed to come on after meals, particularly if you had had a large meal out with alcohol. It was always worse on lying flat and you used to have to get up in the night and walk around until the pain subsided. The sensation could be described as a burning. The pain was often associated with a feeling of generalized bloating in the abdomen. The symptoms seemed to have eased off over the past couple of years.

You have been otherwise fit and well and have never taken any regular medication other than Gaviscon. You have never had surgery. If asked, you remember that about 5 years ago, your GP sent you for a camera test down into your stomach. You were told you had something called 'Barrett's Oesophagus' although you did not understand what it meant.

You ask the candidate if this was related to his current problem. You have no allergies.

You have been a smoker since your teenage years, smoking 5-10 per day. You drink occasional alcohol only since it always seemed to make your heartburn worse.

If asked about breathing difficulties or cough, you mention only that you have always had a dry, tickly cough which had been looked into by your GP but no cause was ever found.

Examiner Instructions:

A 68-year-old man has been referred to the surgical registrar on call by his GP with severe dysphagia. The foundation year doctor has been asked to take the initial history and summarise their findings.

After 6 minutes stop the candidate and ask them to 'please summarise your findings, including a differential diagnosis and immediate management plan' for 2 minutes.

Please follow the mark sheet and grade appropriately.

Marksheet: Dysphagia

Task	Achieved	Not Achieved
Wash hands & Introduces self		
Clarifies who they are speaking to		
Elicits presenting complaint		
Offers reassurance and calms patient		
History of presenting complaint		
Explores what the patient means by 'difficulty swallowing'		
Explores associated symptoms		
Asks whether regurgitated food appears digested or as swallowed and how soon it occurs after eating.		
Enquires about relationship between chest pain and laying flat		
Explores differentials – asks about pain		
Enquires about the timeline of symptoms		
Explores differentials – asks about red flags of malignancy		
Asks about past medical & surgical history		
Asks about Drug History, allergies		
Specifically asks about over the counter reflux remedies		
Ask about Family History & Social History		
Enquires about previous investigations including endoscopy		
Explains without using medical jargon how gastro-oesophageal reflux can lead to cell changes in the oesophagus and dysphagia		
Summarises history concisely		
Correctly identifies likely diagnosis of oesophageal cancer top of differentials, name three more		
Examiner's Global Mark	/5	
Actor/Helper Global Mark	/5	
Total	/30	

Learning Points:

Gastro-oesophageal reflux is one of the most important differentials for chest pain. You should familiarise yourself with the key features of chest pain for various differentials. The systemic features of weight loss and anorexia along with the progressive dysphagia to solids and liquids makes malignancy the most worrying differential here.

It is good practice when taking a history of a patient presenting with a specific symptom such as chest pain to consider at least three differential diagnoses: the most common, ie GORD, the one not to miss, ie ACS, and a rare but serious other, ie dissecting thoracic aneurysm.

Most patients present with a vague complaint such a 'difficulty breathing', 'difficulty swallowing' or 'feeling dizzy'. It is essential to use open questions at the beginning of your history to explore what exactly the patient means by these terms before narrowing your questions to include or exclude your differential diagnosis.

11. Right upper quadrant abdominal pain

Student vignette

An overweight Caucasian 45 year old woman has been referred to the surgical take by her GP with abdominal pain.

You are the foundation year doctor on the surgical team and have been asked to take the initial history and then summarise your findings back to the surgical registrar on-call.

After 6 minutes the examiner will stop you and ask you to summarise back your findings, suggest your differential diagnoses and your initial management plan.

Actor Instructions:

You are a 45-year-old woman named Lisa, who saw her GP this morning with severe pain in the top and right parts of your abdomen. The pain started gradually yesterday and is steadily worsening. It is a constant sharp pain radiating round to the back and into your shoulder.

You have been feeling unwell, with nausea, reduced appetite and fever too. The pain is much worse when you take a deep breath, cough or sneeze and improves on lying still. It is now a severe pain and you are asking for analgesia.

If asked specifically: In the previous months you have been noticing pains in the same area, after eating, lasting a few hours. It did seem worse after eating fatty foods and on occasion you felt pain in the Right shoulder.

You are otherwise fit and well, with no drug allergies. Your GP has been advising you to lose weight for the past few years. You smoke 5 cigarettes a year. You do not drink in the week but have 1-2 bottles of wine each at the weekend with friends.

Your older sister had her gallbladder removed 7 years ago; there are otherwise no medical problems in the family.

You have had no chest pain, no difficulty breathing, no change in your bowel habit and no problems passing urine. You are worried you are going to need an operation.

Examiner Instructions:

An overweight Caucasian 45 year old woman has been referred to the surgical take by her GP with abdominal pain. The foundation year doctor has been asked to take the initial history and summarise their findings.

After 6 minutes stop the candidate and ask them to 'please summarise your findings, including a differential diagnosis and immediate management plan' for 2 minutes.

Please follow the mark sheet and grade appropriately.

Marksheet: Right upper quadrant pain

Task	Achieved	Not Achieved
Wash hands & Introduces self		
Clarifies who they are speaking to		
Elicits presenting complaint		
Offers reassurance and calms patient		
History of presenting complaint		
Explores differentials – asks about pain (SOCRATES)		
Explores associated symptoms		
Pain after fatty foods		
Pain radiating to the shoulder tip or scapula		
Explores differentials – asks about pain		
Explores differentials – asks prior vomiting		
Rule out symptoms of obstructive jaundice		
Asks about past medical & surgical history		
Asks about Drug History, allergies		
Ask about Family History & Social History		
Explores patient's Ideas, Concerns and Expectations		
Summarises history concisely		
Explains further immediate management (Approach using an ABCDE technique)		
Acute cholecystitis top of differentials, name three more		
Clinical Sign- Positive Murphy's sign (accept correct description of sign without name)		
Examiner's Global Mark	/5	
Actor/Helper Global Mark	/5	
Total	/30	

Learning Points:

Practice presenting and summarizing your history in systematic manner, this will help you as an F1 next year and avoid you losing precious time during the exam. Start by offering a single sentence summary/overview of the main issues.

This is a 45 year old woman with severe RUQ, fever and a history of pain suggestive of biliary colic.

Your next sentence or two (max) should highlight the other important positives of the history,

She has been unwell for 24hrs with pain radiating to the shoulder and worse on deep inspiration. She has multiple risk factors for biliary colic and has a positive family history.

Provide any important negatives in your next sentence.

She denies any jaundice and has not had any previous surgery or known gallstones.

Finally conclude with your impression, differential diagnosis and/or next steps (if asked).

This patient probably has acute cholecystitis but we should also exclude pancreatitis as she is a binge-drinker.

Know the key features of the possible differential diagnoses. The examiners aren't here to trick you but to test if you are able to recognize key important conditions. Here is a quick guide to the differential diagnosis of upper abdominal pain.

Biliary Colic- 5 Fs (female, fat, forty, fair and fertile), intermittent pain, onset few hours after eating, lasts 1-3 hrs, radiates round to the back. Worse after fatty meal.

Acute cholecystitis- hx of biliary colic previously, similar but more severe pain last longer (over 6hrs) associated with fever and general malaise

Ascending cholangitis- hx of gallstones, cholecystectomy or ERCP, Charcot's triad of RUQ, fever and jaundice. Pts often septic.

Pancreatitis- hx of risk factors (GETSMASHED), epigastric pain radiating to the back, nausea, diarrhea or vomiting + malaise.

12. Peripheral Vascular Disease

Student vignette

A 68-year-old male has presented to hospital unable to move his left leg.

You are the foundation year doctor on the general surgical team and have been asked to take the initial history and then summarise your findings back to the team.

After 6 minutes the examiner will stop you and ask you to summarise back your findings, suggest your differential diagnoses and your initial management plan.

Actor Instructions:

You are a 68-year-old gentleman named James, who has come to hospital unable to move your left leg. You are able to move your hip but cannot move it at all at the knee or below. This started suddenly, 4 hours ago and you have not been able to move it at all during this time. Your leg is very painful throughout the entirety of the lower leg. The pain does not radiate anywhere and is a very severe, constant pain rating 10/10. Your pain is so severe that unless the candidate offers you pain relief you should be obstructive with giving the history until this is offered.

The appearance of your leg has changed as well. It looks paler in comparison to the other side. However not mottled. When you have touched your leg it has felt very cold. You think your leg has gone numb but it is hard to tell due to the amount of pain.

You cannot walk at all. Before this happened you could walk about 50 metres but would have to stop and take a break due to pain in your calves. Once you rested for a while these pains would disappear.

You have multiple co-morbidities. You have had 2 TIAs (mini-strokes) in the past. You suffer from high cholesterol, type 2 diabetes, ischaemic heart disease and high blood pressure.

You take the following medications:

Amlodipine 10mgOD, Metformin 500mg BD, Bisoprolol 5mg OD, Ramipril 5mg OD, Aspirin 75mg OD, Atorvastatin 10mg ON, GTN spray PRN

You smoke 20 cigarettes a day, drink 1 pint of lager a day on average and live alone.

Examiner Instructions:

A 68 year old gentleman has come to the hospital unable to move his left leg.

The foundation year doctor has been asked to take the initial history and summarise their findings.

After 6 minutes stop the candidate and ask them to 'please summarise your findings, including a differential diagnosis and immediate management plan' for 2 minutes.

Please follow the mark sheet and grade appropriately.

Marksheet: Leg pain

Task	Achieved	Not Achieved
Wash hands & Introduces self		
Clarifies who they are speaking to		
Elicits presenting complaint		
Offers pain relief promptly		
Explores patient's pain (SOCRATES)		
Explores appearance of the leg		
Elicits leg feels cold		
Elicits previous symptoms of peripheral vascular disease		
History of claudication		
Asks about peripheral risk factors: TIA/IHD/High cholesterol		
Asks about past medical & surgical history		
Asks about Drug History, allergies		
Ask about Family History & Social History		
Smoking History		
Exercise Tolerance		
Summarises history concisely		
Provides differential diagnoses (name three)		
Explains further immediate management ABCDE, full neurovascular examination		
Recognises Acute Limb Ischaemia		
Mentions likely emboli due to acute onset and plan for urgent emergency surgery (limb salvage)		
Examiner's Global Mark	/5	
Actor/Helper Global Mark	/5	
Total	/30	

Learning Points:

Acute limb ischaemia is a surgical emergency characterised by the '6 P's' Pain!!!! paralysis, paraesthesia, pulseless, pale and perishingly cold. These findings can be picked up in any clinical setting (primary or secondary care) so there should be no excuse for not considering this diagnosis early and directing the patient to the appropriate vascular opinion.

The majority of cases are caused by a thrombus of an atheroma or by an embolus in those prone to clot formation. Acute scenarios are commonly due to an embolus and atrial fibrillation

Critical ischaemia can be defined by the presence of ischaemic pain at rest, or tissue loss in the form of gangrene or ulcers. It is consistent with an ABPI of < 0.4. Candidates should reacquaint themselves with the method to perform an ABPI.

13. Haematuria

Student vignette

You are the foundation year doctor attached to the GP practice and have been asked to see a 75 year old male who is complaining of intermittent haematuria.

You have been asked to take the initial history and then summarise your findings back to your GP Consultant.

After 6 minutes the examiner will stop you and ask you to summarise back your findings, suggest your differential diagnoses and your initial management plan.

Actor Instructions

You are a 75-year-old gentleman named Jonathan, who has noticed blood in your urine. There is no pain. You don't have any pain but are worried that you may be bleeding internally and so you have come to your GP. You noticed the blood a couple of weeks ago when your urine started getting darker than usual. The urine cleared up over the next day and so you took no notice of it. A couple of days later however you noticed it again and called the GP practice for an urgent appointment. You have never experienced anything like this before. Now you have noticed red clots and are feeling lightheaded.

You have had problems with your waterworks in the past. Reduced capacity to hold onto your urine and having to wake up middle of the night to urinate several times. You have also noticed that your stream is not as strong as it used to be with terminal dribbling. You do not have any other medical problems and are not on any regular medications. You have no allergies that you know of. You live at home with your wife and dog. In the past you used to work in textile manufacturing company. You do smoke and drink alcohol occasionally.

Examiner Instructions

A 75-year-old man has presented to the GP practice complaining of blood in his urine. The foundation year doctor has been asked to take the initial history and summarise their findings.

After 6 minutes stop the candidate and ask them to 'please summarise your findings, including a differential diagnosis and immediate management plan' for 2 minutes.

Please follow the mark sheet and grade appropriately.

Marksheet: Haematuria

Task	Achieved	Not Achieved
Wash hands & Introduces self		
Clarifies who they are speaking to		
Elicits presenting complaint		
Offers reassurance and calms patient		
History of presenting complaint		
Explores Heamaturia		
Explores associated symptoms		
Explores differentials – asks about pain (SOCRATES)		
Asks about storage symptoms- urgency, nocturia, frequency		
Asks about voiding symptoms- hesitancy, poor stream, terminal dribbling, incomplete voiding, dysuria		
Explores differentials – asks about red flags of malignancy		
Asks about previous occupational history		
Asks about past medical & surgical history		
Asks about Drug History, allergies		
Ask about Family History & Social History		
Summarises history concisely		
Explains further immediate management (Approach using an ABCDE technique)		
Offers to examine abdomen and perform Rectal Examination		
Bladder cancer top of differentials, name three more		
Frank haematuria, insertion of 3 way catheter and actively suction of clots with syringe		
Examiner's Global Mark	/5	
Actor/Helper Global Mark	/5	
Total	/30	

Learning Points:

When assessing a patient with haematuria remember that the most severe cause is cancer of the urinary tract but the most common cause in men is BPH.

Remember that painless haematuria can occur anywhere in the urinary tract not just in the bladder.

Assessment of this patient will include imaging of the upper tracts (ideally with a CT IVU), a flexible cystoscopy and in men a DRE and PSA (take PSA before performing DRE).

14. Testicular Swelling

Student vignette

You have been asked to see a 27-year-old male who is complaining of a dull ache in his left testicle.

You are the foundation year doctor on the urology team and have been asked to take the initial history and then summarise your findings back to the surgical registrar on-call.

After 6 minutes the examiner will stop you and ask you to summarise back your findings, suggest your differential diagnoses and your initial management plan.

Actor Instructions

You are a 27-year-old man named Martin who works as an actor in a theatre company. You have come to hospital complaining of a dull ache in the back of your left testis. There is no radiation but you have noticed that your left testis is larger than your right one. You feel a dragging sensation on the left side when you stand up. This ache has been on-going for 3 month and has only moderately improved with simple analgesia.

You can't remember any injury to your testis however do note that you have been feeling feverish recently and having night sweats. You have normal waterworks and bowel habits. Your mother has noticed that you're becoming thin and your clothes do not fit as well.

On further questioning you do remember your mother telling you that you had problems with your testes as a child and had an operation to "bring the testes down". You have had no other operations and are normally fit and well.

You do not take any regular medication and have no allergies. You are a smoker (smoke 10-15/day) and drink regular alcohol. You are sexually active but have no stable partner.

Examiner Instructions:

A 27-year-old male has presented to the department complaining of a dull ache in his left testicle. The foundation year doctor has been asked to take the initial history and summarise their findings.

After 6 minutes stop the candidate and ask them to 'please summarise your findings, including a differential diagnosis and immediate management plan' for 2 minutes.

Please follow the mark sheet and grade appropriately.

Marksheet: Testicular pain

Task	Achieved	Not Achieved
Wash hands & Introduces self		
Clarifies who they are speaking to		
Elicits presenting complaint		
Offers reassurance and calms patient		
History of presenting complaint		
Explores patient's pain (SOCRATES)		
Explores associated symptoms- fever, rigors, urinary symptoms		
Asks about constitutional symptoms (lymphadenopathy, night sweats, weight loss)		
Asks about previous trauma		
Sexual health History		
Foreign travel History		
Asks about past medical & surgical history		
Asks about Drug History, allergies		
Ask about Family History & Social History		
Summarises history concisely		
Suggest performing abdominal, testicular and rectal examination		
Explains further immediate management		
Testicular cancer top of differentials, name three more		
Suggest urine dip, USS testes		
Name the tumour markers for testicular cancer		
Examiner's Global Mark	/5	
Actor/Helper Global Mark	/5	
Total	/30	

Learning Points:

Testicular cancer is usually a disease of the young have a high index of suspicion in patients with longstanding testicular pain particularly if they have a history of undescended testes. Testicular cancer can occur at any age but is most common between the ages of 15 and 40 years with testicular tumours the most common malignancy in men aged between 20 and 35 years.

A swollen high rising testis should give you a suspicion of testicular torsion. In this case urgent exploration is needed without delay for imaging.

An ultrasound scan of the testis is first line imaging to image any testicular lump however remember that an ultrasound can not rule out a testicular torsion.

15. Loin to Groin Pain

Student vignette

A 41-year-old male has been brought into Emergency Department by ambulance complaining of sudden onset flank pain.

You are the foundation year doctor on the surgical team and have been asked to take the initial history and then summarise your findings back to the surgical registrar on-call.

After 6 minutes the examiner will stop you and ask you to summarise back your findings, suggest your differential diagnoses and your initial management plan.

Actor Instructions:

You will be in visible distress during the history taking. Unable to get comfortable and roll around on the bed until your doctor prescribes/offers you strong pain relief during history taking.

You are a 41-year-old male called James, who works as a project manager in construction. This morning you experienced sudden onset severe right flank pain radiating to your back and down to your groin and scrotum. This pain is like nothing you have felt before and you felt feverish, nauseated and vomiting earlier this morning. The pain comes in waves.

You have had no change in bowel habit however you note that it is particularly uncomfortable passing urine. You have tried taking some paracetamol to no effect. You are finding it difficult to keep still with no particular position offering you any relief.

You do not have any other medical problems and are not on any regular medications. You have no allergies that you know of. Within your family history your mother suffered from hyperparathyroidism. You live at home with your wife and three kids and are generally well otherwise.

Examiner Instructions:

A 41-year-old male has been brought into Emergency Department by ambulance complaining of sudden onset flank pain. The foundation year doctor has been asked to take the initial history and summarise their findings.

After 6 minutes stop the candidate and ask them to 'please summarise your findings, including a differential diagnosis and immediate management plan' for 2 minutes.

Please follow the mark sheet and grade appropriately.

Marksheet:Loin to groin pain

Task	Achieved	Not Achieved
Wash hands & Introduces self		
Clarifies who they are speaking to		
Elicits presenting complaint		
Offers reassurance and calms patient		
Offer patient pain relief		
History of presenting complaint		
Explores patient's pain (SOCRATES)		
Explores associated symptoms- fever, rigors		
Comment on whether patient has testicular pain		
Asks about diet- high protein/ oxalate rich foods, fluid intake		
Asks about past medical & surgical history		
Asks about Drug History, allergies		
Ask about Family History & Social History		
Summarises history concisely		
Explains further immediate management (Approach using an ABCDE technique)		
Renal colic top of differentials, name three more, including AAA		
Mentions this is an emergency & resuscitation		
Understand importance of urgent escalation if patient is septic. i.e. urgent relief of blockage		
Urine dipstick, IVI, IV Antibiotics, Catheter		
Mention CTKUB gold standard investigation		
Examiner's Global Mark	/5	
Actor/Helper Global Mark	/5	
Total	/30	

Learning Points:

Assessing and dealing with pain should be a mandatory task for the clinician at the beginning of every consultation. Check a pain score and then remember to re review that the analgesia has had an effect.

Many cases of renal colic with proven stones can be left for the stone to pass naturally. Take note if there is unremitting pain, fever suggesting superimposed infection, or newly deranged renal function and hydronephrosis.

Repeated episodes of renal calculi may indicate an underlying metabolic disease (primary hyperparathyroidism, cystinuria, hyperoxaluria) and these aetiologies should be considered when patients return to outpatient clinic after the first episode.

16. Neck Swelling

Student vignette

A 40-year-old female has attended your GP practice with new persistent swelling in her neck.

You are the foundation year doctor and have been asked to take the initial history and then summarise your findings back to your GP Consultant.

After 6 minutes the examiner will stop you and ask you to summarise back your findings, suggest your differential diagnoses and your initial management plan.

Actor instructions:

You are a 40-year-old lady called Jasmine, who has been feeling generally run down for some time. You noticed a swelling in your neck several days ago and feel that it has slowly been enlarging since then. It is painless but is starting to affect your appearance. You haven't noticed any lumps elsewhere in your body.

You began to feel unusually tired and lethargic approximately 3 months ago when you were rehearsing for a new role on a television show. You then noticed finding it increasingly difficult to concentrate on learning your lines. You also think you may have put on some weight in the last 2 months even though your diet is unchanged. Generally you have a few more aches and pains when attempting to move across the stage and have started wearing a jacket to work when previously you wouldn't have.

Prior to all of this starting you had been very fit and well. You have had no previous medical problems other than having your appendix removed as a child.

In terms of family history your mother has Diabetes but you don't know of any other familial illnesses. You have no drug allergies and are not on any regular medications. You smoke 5 cigarettes per day and drink two glasses of wine 2-3 times per week.

You are very concerned about what might be going on as it is having significant impact on your life and your ability to do your job. If asked about your concerns you are very worried that it might be cancer and feel very sensitive about this now as one of your best friends recently died with cancer.

Examiner's Instructions:

A 40-year-old female has attended your GP practice with new persistent swelling in her neck. The foundation year doctor has been asked to take the initial history and summarise their findings.

After 6 minutes stop the candidate and ask them to 'please summarise your findings, including a differential diagnosis and immediate management plan' for 2 minutes.

Please follow the mark sheet and grade appropriately.

Marksheet: Neck Lump

Task	Achieved	Not Achieved
Wash hands & Introduces self		
Clarifies who they are speaking to		
Elicits presenting complaint		
Offers reassurance and calms patient		
History of presenting complaint		
In regards to swelling: when was it noticed/change in size, colour		
Explores associated symptoms		
Explores differentials – asks about pain (SOCRATES)		
Ask if she has noticed any other lumps		
Explores differentials – asks about red flags of malignancy		
Systemic features: weight gain, sensitive to temperature, aches		
Asks about past medical & surgical history		
Asks about Drug History, allergies		
Ask about Family History & Social History		
Summarises history concisely		
Asks patient open question about her concerns		
Responds empathetically towards her		
Hashimoto thyroiditis top of differentials, name three more		
Mentions performing full ENT Examination and nasoendoscopy		
Management – triple assessment, Ex, USS, FNA and thyroid profile blood test		
Examiner's Global Mark	/5	
Actor/Helper Global Mark	/5	
Total	/30	

Learning Points:

Every lump in the neck is managed in a triple assessment clinic (examination, ultrasound imaging with FNA cytology)

Goitres can be caused by conditions leading to both under and over activity of the thyroid gland. The clues will be in the History that you take.

The most common cause of goitre worldwide is iodine deficiency that leads to 90% of cases and can lead to hypothyroidism.

17. Breast Lump

Student vignette

A 49-year-old female has attended her General Practice clinic with a lump in her right breast.

You are the foundation year doctor and have been asked to take the initial history and then summarise your findings back to the GP Consultant.

After 6 minutes the examiner will stop you and ask you to summarise back your findings, suggest your differential diagnoses and your initial management plan.

Actor Instructions:

You are a 49-year-old lady, very anxious, complaining of having a 3-month history of right breast ache and bloody nipple discharge.

Over the last month, you have noticed a lump in the right breast; increasing in size, irregular shape of your breast with crusty red skin changes. As well as lower dull backache and decrease in appetite.

Only give this information if asked directly. You have been losing weight unintentionally over the last month.

You suffered from early periods and are now menopausal.

You do not have any other medical problems and are not on any regular medications. You have no allergies that you know of.

You are fit and active but smoke 20 cigarettes a day with occasionally drink alcohol

You are very concerned about what might be going on as it is having significant impact on your life. You have been too scared to seek medical advice. Your sister and mother have suffered from breast cancer.

Examiner Instructions:

A 49-year-old female has attended her General Practice clinic with a lump in her right breast. The foundation year doctor has been asked to take the initial history and summarise their findings.

After 6 minutes stop the candidate and ask them to 'please summarise your findings, including a differential diagnosis and immediate management plan' for 2 minutes. Please follow the mark sheet and grade appropriately.

Marksheet:Breast Lump

Task:	Achieved	Not Achieved
Wash hands & Introduces self		
Clarifies who they are speaking to		
Elicits presenting complaint		
Offers reassurance and calms patient		
History of presenting complaint		
Ask about red flags- Lump, sudden increase in size, skin changes		
Ask about red flags- Nipple inversion/discharge/skin changes/ulceration		
Ask about pain (SOCRATES)		
Associated weight loss and back pain		
Gynecological History		
Asks about past medical & surgical history		
Asks about Drug History, allergies		
Ask about Family History & Social History		
Summarises history concisely		
Show empathy		
Address Ideas, concerns and expectations		
Breast cancer top of differentials, name three more		
Discuss 2 week referral to breast surgical one-stop clinic		
Triple assessment (examination, mammogram and core biopsy)		
Discuss Surgical and medical management for breast cancer		
Examiner's Global Mark	/5	
Actor / Helper's Global Mark	/5	
Total Station Mark	/30	

Learning Points:

Every patient with a breast lump should be referred to the one-stop breast clinic for triple assessment (examination, imaging, core biopsy)and review by a specialist.

Remember to ask about relevant gynaecological history such as age of menarche, menopause, parity, breastfeeding, contraceptive and hormone replacement therapy.

Have a systematic approach to history taking, covering the red flags for breast disease:
> Breast lump
> Nipple eczema or retraction
> Skin distortion
> Persisting, intense unilateral pain

18. Pre-Operative Assessment of the High Risk Surgical patient

Student vignette

A 78-year-old male with significant co-morbidities has attended the pre-operative assessment clinic. He is due to have a Hartmann's for a sigmoid colon tumour. He is managed in the community for chronic obstructive pulmonary disease (COPD).

You are the foundation year doctor on the surgical team and have been asked to take the initial history and then summarise your findings back to the surgical registrar on-call.

After 6 minutes the examiner will stop you and ask you to summarise back your findings, suggest your differential diagnoses and your initial management plan.

Actor Instructions

You are a 78-year-old man named Gerald, who has presented with a new diagnosis of sigmoid colon cancer confirmed on your recent CT Scan and tissue histology. You have agreed to have surgery.

You are a gentleman who does not leave the house.

You have type 2 diabetes mellitus, hypertension and COPD (chronic obstructive pulmonary disease). A specialist nurse in the community currently manages your lung disease.

Your regular medications consist of metformin 1g twice daily, Gliclazide 40mg once daily, Ramipril 2.5mg once a day and you take a range of inhalers. You have no allergies that you know of.

You have previously been told that your COPD is poorly controlled as you continue to smoke between 20-30 cigarettes per day. You are unable to walk further than a flight of stairs without becoming breathless, however you are not breathless at rest in a chair.

You currently receive a three times daily care package which includes cleaning of the house and currently feel this will be sufficient post operatively. You have no family who live nearby. You are concerned regarding how you get back to health after the operation and whether any support in hospital will be provided to get you back to your feet.

You are unsure why you have had to attend this meeting today as the surgeon has already informed you that the operation will be going ahead.

Examiner Instructions

A 78-year-old male with significant co-morbidities has attended the pre-operative assessment clinic. He is due to have a Hartmann's for a sigmoid colon tumour. He is managed in the community for chronic obstructive pulmonary disease (COPD). The foundation year doctor has been asked to take the initial history and summarise their findings.

After 6 minutes stop the candidate and ask them to 'please summarise your findings, including a differential diagnosis and immediate management plan' for 2 minutes.

Please follow the mark sheet and grade appropriately.

Marksheet: Pre op assessment

Task	Achieved	Not Achieved
Wash hands & Introduces self		
Clarifies who they are speaking to		
Offers reassurance and calms patient		
Elicits history from patient in a concise manner		
Asks about reasoning for surgery		
Asks about current symptoms		
Enquires regarding current management of condition		
Asks about co-morbidity		
Specific focus on cardiovascular disease and symptoms (hypertension, congestive heart failure, diabetes, valvular disease)		
Current cardiovascular disease treatments		
Directly questions exercise tolerance		
Thorough review of alcohol, smoking and drug status		
Asks about Drug History, allergies		
Asks about past medical & surgical history		
Identifies patients risk (low, intermediate, high)		
Informs patient of the risks associated with surgery (early, intermediate and late)		
Ask about Family History & Social History		
Identifies ideas, concerns and expectations		
Summarises history concisely		
Post operative care – Physiotherapy, occupational therapy, assisted discharge, district nurse involvement		
Examiner's Global Mark	/5	
Actor/Helper Global Mark	/5	
Total	/30	

Learning Points:

Pre-operative assessment is a specialty with growing emphasis toward shared decision making and patient choice. The patient must understand the risks and benefits of the procedures. This can be informed to the patient in a manner using a risk stratification score such as P-POSSUM.

Time must be taken to establish the patient's co-morbidities along with a discussion of how any of these risk factors could be optimised to allow the anaesthetist, surgeon and ultimately the patient the best chance of success.

Understanding activities of daily living, and the support the patient currently receives and may require post operatively is also becoming increasingly important when considering patients care post operatively

Chapter Two

Communication Scenarios

19. Blood Transfusion Discussion

Student vignette

You are the foundation year doctor on a surgical firm. Gloria is a 72-year-old woman who has been admitted for an elective anterior resection for a sigmoid cancer. She is anaemic (haemoglobin of 75g/dL) and requires a blood transfusion prior to the operation.

She has asked to discuss issues she has related to receiving a blood transfusion.

Actor Instructions:

You are Gloria a 72 year old lady who has been admitted to hospital for a planned operation to remove a cancer from your large bowel. You were briefly informed by the admitting doctor that you were anaemic and may need a blood transfusion prior to any operation. The nursing staff has informed you blood has been ordered and prescribed to be given to you.

You are unhappy that although the admitting doctor suggested this plan, it was never confirmed.

You are worried about the risks of blood transfusions and are particularly concerned about the prospect of hepatitis, a disease you have read can be transmitted in blood transfusions. You are eager to know of any other alternatives to blood transfusions so as to avoid any complications.

You are unaware of the indications for transfusion and as far as you are concerned feel fine and therefore think it an unnecessary requirement prior to your operation.

You should continue to be resistant to the suggestion of a blood transfusion unless the candidate gives good reason for its administration and reassures you that the risks of infection and other transfusion reactions are outweighed by the benefits of being optimized before a major operation.

Examiner Instructions:

A **72**-year-old woman has been admitted for an elective anterior resection for a sigmoid cancer. She is anaemic (haemoglobin of 75g/dL) and requires a blood transfusion prior to the operation. The candidate is required to assess the patient's knowledge of their needs of a transfusion in the context of their operation. They should also ask for specific concerns related to this and their expectations of the consultation

The candidate should explain the risks and benefits of transfusions in a well-structured manner.

The candidate should offer alternatives to transfusions (iron infusions and the use of cell savers intraoperatively).

The candidate should summarise and check the patient's understanding.
The candidate should offer reassurance and not press the patient if she chooses to opt against a transfusion in the context of all relevant factors.

Please follow the mark sheet and grade appropriately.

Marksheet: Blood transfusion

Task:	Achieved	Not Achieved
Introduces self		
Clarifies who they are speaking		
Elicits knowledge from patient		
Asks about concerns		
Asks about expectations of consultation		
Explains transfusion requirement in anaemia		
Explains transfusion requirement pre-operatively		
Explains infective risks of blood transfusions		
Explains reaction risks of transfusion reactions		
Explains the process of blood grouping to minimise possibility of immune reactions		
Explains the risk of fluid overload		
Explains Cell saver alternative		
Explains iron infusion alternative		
Checks patient understanding		
Evaluates patient's decision on which management they prefer in a non pressured manner		
Summarises appropriately		
Thanks the patient and closes appropriately		
Demonstrates empathy		
Explains in a clear structured manner		
Offers reading material on blood transfusions		
Examiner's Global Mark	/5	
Actor / Helper's Global Mark	/5	
Total Station Mark	/30	

Learning Points:

Always check knowledge, address concerns and expectations of the patient. Most scenarios can be dealt with in a more efficient and collaborative manner if their ICE is examined early and discussed openly.

The purpose of the station and most real life clinical scenarios is not to convince the patient to accept a blood transfusion but to educate them to make the best informed decision.

If the patient still wishes to not be transfused do not take this as a failure – all you can do is give them all the information they can make a decision with. If you feel the patient does not have capacity to make a decision then a formal assessment of capacity needs to be documented and your seniors informed immediatey.

20. Conversation on DNAR

Student vignette

You are the foundation year doctor on the general surgery team looking after Daryl an 89-year-old man with Alzheimer's disease, End stage heart failure and chronic kidney disease. He has been admitted with CT confirmed acute ischaemic bowel. He is unsuitable for surgery and has been deteriorating. His family has been informed that he will not undergo surgery and sadly he is approaching the end of his life.

You have been asked by your registrar to discuss a do not resuscitate order with his daughter Denise (his next of kin) in the context of his prognosis, comorbidities and his worsening confusion.

Actor Instructions:

You are Denise the daughter of Daryl an 89-year-old gentleman who normally lives in a nursing home

He has been admitted to hospital unwell with severe abdominal pain. The admitting teams have done investigations (including a scan) which have revealed him to have suffered bowel ischaemia. They have explained that this is a catastrophic event which he will not survive and you have seen him deteriorate from being his normal but confused self in the days before admission to being minimally responsive in the emergency departments' resus area.

Although you know he is not a fit man – he has multiple health problems including Alzheimer's, heart failure and kidney disease he is happily confused and has intermittent lucid intervals when he recognizes family. You understand that he is dying but you are shocked he has gone downhill so quickly and find this distressing.

You have never had any conversations with your father about what he would want if his heart stopped (whether he would want chest compressions).

You do not know what a do not attempt resuscitation (DNAR) order entails. You are frightened that not having an operation means that the medical team will do nothing for your father. You are particularly concerned that he will suffer pain. Your mother died in hospital and suffered with severe pain and nausea in the final stages of her life and you would hate to see him suffer the same fate.

The candidate is likely to confirm you understand the current clinical diagnosis and likely course of your father before attempting to discuss resuscitation. You should focus on your concerns about this and be resistant to discussing resuscitation before this is addressed.

Examiner Instructions:

The candidate has been asked to discuss the resuscitation status of Daryl Davies and 89-year-old gentleman (who is currently deteriorating due to acute gut ischaemia) with his daughter.

This scenario is designed to assess the candidates' manner in communicating about a sensitive subject with the family of a dying patient. The Candidate is likely to assess the daughters' knowledge of the scenario and their worries about what her father will encounter as he deteriorates. From this initial foundation the concerns of the daughter can be allayed and provide a direction from which the discussion of resuscitation status can be approached appropriately.

The scenario should be handled with subtlety and sensitivity.

Please follow the mark sheet and grade appropriately.

Marksheet: DNAR

Task:	Achieved	Not Achieved
Candidate introduces self		
Candidate confirms patients daughter's identity		
Candidate explains role		
Candidate volunteers area of privacy/private room to have discussion		
Candidate asks if daughter would like to have another family member present or member of nursing staff		
Candidate assesses daughters knowledge of the situation		
Candidate explores and acknowledges daughters concerns		
Candidate explores daughter expectations of consultation		
Candidate relays back their clinical understanding of problem		
Candidate explores daughters understanding of DNAR		
Candidate explains DNAR		
Candidate addresses concerns of father being in pain by explaining priority of symptom control		
Candidate suggests input of macmillan/palliative care teams		
Candidate summarises discussion		
Candidate closes appropriately		
Candidate approaches discussion in structured manner		
Candidate listens actively		
Candidate allows appropriate silences and pauses		
Candidate demonstrates empathy and sensitivity		
Candidate offers reading materials		
Examiner's Global Mark	/5	
Actor / Helper's Global Mark	/5	
Total Station Mark	/30	

Learning Points:

Difficult discussions should be had on the patient's/relative's terms – their concerns should be at the centre of this. If they are addressed the clinician can communicate their agenda clearly. Often the message to be conveyed is not the stumbling block but instead the way to say it becomes the issues.

Honesty and openness in the osce or real life is always a good place to start. If you don't know all the answers say this openly but offer to pursue them and return with a senior to clarify.

A focus on communication skills will always be reflected in the mark schemes of these stations so ICE, summarise, confirm knowledge repeatedly if necessary to ensure actor comfort at all times.

21. Assessing a patient- Post-operative confusion

Student vignette

You are the foundation year doctor in the in general surgery. Jack is an 80-year-old man who underwent an emergency repair of an incarcerated inguinal hernia 2 days ago. Prior to surgery he lived independently with his wife with no medical history apart from hypertension. The ward nursing staff has contacted your team because he is allegedly confused. Your registrar has asked you to obtain a history to the best of your abilities in order to assess their mental status.

After 6 minutes the examiner will stop you and ask you to summarise back your findings, suggest your differential diagnoses and your initial management plan.

Actor Instructions:

You are Jack an 80-year-old man who had an emergency repair of a hernia 2 days ago. The nursing staff believes you are confused and have asked one of the foundation doctors to assess you.

You believe you are at the local golf club, not in hospital. You believe it is 1958. You assume the gentleman who speaks to you is a young club member and not a doctor as he may suggest. The doctor is likely to ask you about physical symptoms such as pain and shortness of breath however you maintain a disengaged affect with little cooperation with questioning. They may go on to ask specific questions about your age, date of birth, the time and the year. You may find such questions ridiculous and impertinent unless they are proposed in a reassuring and sensitive manner

Initially you are happily confused and this should continue if the doctor attending you maintains a relaxed and reassuring manner. If there are any non-reassuring aspects to their manner or they become frustrated then you may find this confusing and therefore distressing and become increasingly agitated.

The confused affect should continue for the duration of the scenario and is a test of the candidate's stamina in maintaining patience with a floridly confused patient.

Examiner Instructions:

The candidate has been asked to obtain a history/assess the mental status of Jack an 80-year-old gentleman two days after an emergency hernia repair.

The patient will maintain a confused affect throughout the scenario and is likely to cooperate minimally with the candidates questioning/assessment.

The candidate should address/introduce themselves to the patient as normal. They should go on to ask basic screening questions of the patients in terms of symptoms. It will soon become apparent that the patient is confused. The candidate should then attempt to perform an abbreviated mental test.

This is likely to be performed with limited success but all aspects should be attempted.

The candidate should persevere with the patient in order to assess them as fully as possible. This should be done reassuringly, with no element of frustration or pressure on the patient so as not to cause any agitation or confusion.

If the candidate attempts to examine the patient then prompt them that it is a history taking station.
After 6 minutes stop the candidate and ask the following questions for 2 minutes
What AMT score has been achieved?
What are the differentials for the patient's clinical state?
What are the causes of an acute delirium particularly in this patient?
How would you manage this patient?
How would you investigate this patient?

Please follow the mark sheet and grade appropriately.

Marksheet: Post op confusion

Task:	Achieved	Not Achieved
Candidate introduces self		
Candidate confirms patient identity (this may be with a name band)		
Candidate establishes/explains role		
Candidate attempts to ask a symptom screen		
Candidate asks patient age		
Candidate asks patients the current time		
Candidate asks patient the current year		
Candidate asks patient the name of the building they are in		
Candidate asks the patient if they recognize two people/objects		
Candidate asks patient date of birth		
Candidate asks patient date recall question (what date was world war two etc)		
Candidate asks patient name of current monarch		
Candidate asks patient to count back from 20-1.		
Candidate attempts to ask patient to register and recall address (eg 42 west street)		
Candidate summarises discussion		
Candidate closes appropriately		
Candidate approaches discussion in structured manner		
Candidate listens actively		
Candidate allows appropriate silences and pauses		
Candidate demonstrates empathy and sensitivity		
Examiner's Global Mark	/5	
Actor / Helper's Global Mark	/5	
Total Station Mark	/30	

Learning Points:

Delirium is a clinical syndrome which is difficult to define exactly but involves abnormalities of thought, perception and levels of awareness. It typically is of acute onset and intermittent and can exhibit hypo and hyperactive episodes.

Post operatively remember to consider if there is an iatrogenic cause for the acute change - has the patient been prescribed anything that has made them confused. Blood sugars and infection screens can be initiated early to identify a cause.

The AMTS is absolutely key here. Once you have established the patient is confused and there is not much history to be gained, assessment of mental state should be the priority.

22. Consent for Flexible Sigmoidoscopy procedure

Student vignette

You are the foundation year doctor in the surgical assessment unit. John is a 60-year-old man who has been reviewed with intermittent rectal bleeding. He is to be invited back to the endoscopy unit for a flexible sigmoidoscopy to investigate this. This will occur in the next two weeks.

You have been asked by your registrar to explain the procedure 'flexible sigmoidoscopy 'to the patient.

Actor Instructions:

You are John a 60-year-old photographer from London. You have been having intermittent bleeding from your back passage for 2 months and have attended the surgical assessment unit for a flexible sigmoidoscopy. You are extremely concerned that the bleeding may be due to cancer.

You know little about the procedure apart from that it involves a camera and your back passage. You worry that it will be painful, embarrassing and that a camera passing up your back passage could cause damage. You are also anxious that you could have the test and find out that you might have cancer particularly because a friend has recently been diagnosed with colon cancer.

You would appreciate an explanation of the procedure, what benefits and risks there are and what you need to do to prepare and recover from it. If there are any less invasive alternatives you would like to be told about them so that you can know what other options you may be able to choose.
Because of your concerns about cancer you really want to be investigated as soon as possible. You would also appreciate some reading materials so you can look into this further in your own time.

Examiner Instructions:

The candidate has been asked to explain the flexible sigmoidoscopy procedure to a patient, John who is to be referred for this as an outpatient as an urgent two-week referral.

The patient knows nothing of the procedure and wishes to know all about it in terms of what to expect, how he should prepare and what risks and benefits the procedure entails. He is anxious as a friend has been recently diagnosed with colon cancer and he is worried his symptoms may be due to this.

The candidate should establish the patient's knowledge of the procedure and his concerns and expectations of the consultation. From there he should explain the procedure practically and in terms of what risks and benefits it entails. The candidate's explanation should address all concerns and expectations. This should be done in a structured manner to enable better understanding. By the end of the station the candidate should confirm the patient's understanding much like a formal consenting.

If the candidate begins to delve into the patient's symptoms and history in detail please interrupt in order to remind them that the history has been taken and that their role is to explain the investigation only.

The scenario should be handled with subtlety and sensitivity.

Please follow the mark sheet and grade appropriately.

Marksheet: Flexible Sigmoidoscopy

Task:	Achieved	Not Achieved
Candidate introduces him/herself and confirms patient identity		
Candidate explains their role to the patient		
Candidate confirms patient's current understanding, their worries and expectations of the consultation		
Candidate approaches explaining/addressing concerns in a clear structured manner		
Candidate explains that bowel preparation (enema/laxatives) is required		
Candidate explains that the procedure visualizes the rectum and the last portion of the large bowel (appropriate description of the endoscope used)		
Candidate explains general aspects of the procedure (a small camera with a similar width to a little finger with a light source is introduced to the back passage. Images from the camera are seen and assessed by the endoscopist as the procedure is carried out)		
Candidate explains the use of painkillers and/or sedatives to enable procedure and it should not be painful		
Candidate explain that if sedation is used the patient will not be able to drive themselves home and will require a friend/family member to supervise them after the procedure.		
Candidate explains that after the procedure they will be taken to the recovery area		
Candidate explains the benefits of the procedure – visualization of the bowel and acquisition of tissue samples for diagnostic purposes		
Candidate explains that there are risks, specifically bowel perforation, infection and bleeding but that these are rare		
Candidate explains that if polyps are removed there may be further fresh blood from the back passage over 12-24 hours after the procedure.		

Candidate explains that if samples are taken they will be processed in approximately 2 weeks.		
Candidate explains alternatives to flexible sigmoidoscopy, barium enema, ct colonography and briefly their benefits (non invasive) and limitations (no tissue diagnosis).		
Candidate summarises appropriately and prompts further questioning		
Candidate offers reading material		
Candidate demonstrates explanation in clear structured manner		
Candidate listens appropriately		
Candidate demonstrates empathy and sensitivity		
Examiner's Global Mark	/5	
Actor / Helper's Global Mark	/5	
Total Station Mark	/30	

Learning Points:

Explaining procedures and interventions is a common task for the foundation year doctor and so rightly many OSCEs are based around this. Having a structure is important - check understanding thus far, explain indications, contraindications, the location and duration of the procedure, the mechanics of the procedure itself and of course the potential side effects.

If formal written consent is required as per GMC guidelines this should only be done by someone that can actually carry out the procedure themselves. For procedures and interventions that only require verbal consent it is still good practice to explain all the sections above to ensure fully understanding.

Remember that in some situations patients may decline to give consent to a procedure. You may offer them more time, further reading materials and resources and senior to explain further however if they have capacity they are of course allowed to decline to give consent.

23. Breaking Bad News – Operation Cancelled

Student vignette

You are the foundation year doctor on trauma and orthopedics.

Emma is a 53-year-old lady who was admitted with a fracture dislocated right ankle 3 days ago and is awaiting an open reduction internal fixation of this injury. Unfortunately her operation has been cancelled today because of the number and priority of other orthopedic admissions requiring surgery.

Your registrar has asked you to inform Emma that her operation will not happen today.

Actor Instructions:

You are Emma a 53-year-old woman who broke her right ankle 3 days ago whilst walking her dog. You have been waiting for an operation to manage this problem since admission.

This is the second day that you have been made nil by mouth (starved) in order to prepare you for the operation. As such you are hungry and anxious to go to theatre to have the operation. The operation was cancelled late in the day yesterday and the nursing staff that it would happen today assured you.

Aside from the frustration of a late cancellation yesterday you are particularly concerned that delays will affect how your ankle will heal and may leave you permanently disabled. You are also desperate to get home to your dog, as you live alone and he is temporarily staying with a neighbour.

If you were to be informed that the operation was cancelled a second time you would likely be angry and upset that your operation is not considered a priority and that cancellation was not foreseen earlier so that you could have eaten. You may be pacified by explanation that due to the limitations of the trauma operating list mean that urgent cases on children and the elderly have to be prioritized. However if your fears are not allayed you may feel insistent on speaking to a consultant in order to complain.

Examiner Instructions:

Emma is a 53-year-old woman who was admitted 3 days ago with a broken ankle and has been kept nil by mouth for two consecutive days waiting for an operation on this.

The foundation year doctor has been asked to inform her that for a second day her operation will be cancelled. She has been starved for two days and is anxious about long-term disability and her dog at home. The candidate should demonstrate adequate breaking bad news skills in an empathic manner and manage patient's frustrations by listening appropriately before exploring patient concerns and addressing any expectations they are able to.

The scenario should be handled with subtlety and sensitivity.

Please follow the mark sheet and grade appropriately.

Marksheet: Breaking Bad News - cancelled operation

Task:	Achieved	Not Achieved
Candidate introduces self		
Candidate confirmation of patient details		
Candidate explains their role		
Candidate establishes patients current understanding of the situation		
Candidate explores patient's current concerns related to their clinical problem		
Candidate Breaks bad news that operation has been cancelled in empathic manner with signposting/appropriate warning shot		
Candidate allows the patient time to digest the news that operation has been cancelled		
Informs patient that they may now eat and drink		
Explains the nature of emergency theatres and possibility of cancellation appropriately		
Explains that the plan for operation will continue BUT that there may still be a possibility of cancellation on the trauma list		
Candidate suggestion that there may be a possibility of the ankle being treated on a non emergency list but this would have to be arranged at a consultant level		
Candidate offers to discuss with a senior if patient still not happy or has further questions		
Candidate offers advice regarding patient advice and liaison service if patient adamant they wish to complain		
Candidate summarises discussion		
Candidate closes appropriately		
Candidate approaches discussion in a structured, clear manner		
Candidate listens actively		
Candidate allows appropriate silences and pauses		
Candidate demonstrates empathy and sensitivity		
Examiner's Global Mark	/5	
Actor / Helper's Global Mark	/5	
Total Station Mark	/30	

Learning Points:

Inevitably in medicine we will have to deliver news to patients and families that is not welcomed or expected and having a strategy to do this is essential. Like this scenario breaking bad news is not just about the high end scenarios of cancer and end of life but more commonly cancelled operations and delays to investigations and test results.

Silence is your friend. Uninterrupted patients will tend to talk out their frustrations and concerns until they have matters off their chest. These can then be broken down and addressed individually.

Openness and honesty is essential in communication scenarios. if you don't know the answer to a question then offer to find out. Do not lie or cover up any failings and do not be afraid to say you are sorry for the situation that has occurred.

24. The upset relative

Student vignette

You are the foundation year doctor in the surgical assessment unit. Samantha is the 35-year-old mother of Tom a 9-year-old child who is currently being operated on for an emergency splenic rupture. He was with his father when he apparently fell from off his bicycle.

She is very upset and the nursing staff has asked you to speak with her and address her concerns.

Actor Instructions:

You have received a call an hour ago from your ex-husband explaining that your son is being rushed into emergency theatre for a serious injury. You are very upset about the current situation. Extremely anxious and annoyed that a doctor has not called you at once about your son.

You want to see your son now.

You want to know exactly what operation your son is having, complications and is there a risk of him dying?

Treatment after splenectomy for patients, will anything change?

First words should be "why was I not called about this before he was taken for his operation?" If the explanation is good and they apologise explaining it was an emergency then you should then calm down.

You're concerned that whenever your son is with your ex-husband he always ends getting injured. *If prompted, mention that you have gone through a difficult divorce recently, brought about because he is always stressed and drinks too much. Ask what the candidate will do with that information and ask them to keep it to themselves.*

Ask when can you take Tom home? Claim your child is always safe with you

Throughout remain very anxious and wait on silence pauses and warm to candidate if they show empathy.

Examiner Instructions:

The candidate has been asked to hold a conversation with an upset mother who is very concerned that her 9-year-old child Tom has been rushed in for an emergency theatre for splenic rupture.

The candidate should demonstrate adequate breaking bad news skills in an empathic manner and manage patient's frustrations by listening appropriately before exploring patient concerns and addressing any expectations they are able to.

The scenario should be handled with subtlety and sensitivity.

Please follow the mark sheet and grade appropriately.

Marksheet: Upset relative

Task:	Achieved	Not Achieved
Candidate introduces self		
Candidate confirmation of patient details		
Candidate explains their role & expresses sorrow for the situation		
Candidate establishes mother's current understanding of the situation		
Give reason for why she was not contacted		
Candidate explores their current concerns related to their clinical problem		
Candidate Breaks bad news that operation is an emergency signposting/appropriate warning shot		
Candidate allows the mother time to digest the news –severity of the situation		
Explain risks of procedure, avoid medical jargon		
Explore social background, ex-husband and father's drinking issue		
Child safety, child safeguarding procedure in a sensitive way		
Have to involve pediatric team and share information mother has given		
Not to collude with parent		
Discuss post-operative management of patient with splenectomy		
Candidate summarises discussion		
Candidate closes appropriately		
Candidate approaches discussion in a structured, clear manner		
Candidate listens actively and allows appropriate silences and pauses		
Maintains eye contacts, open body language, reassurance		
Candidate demonstrates empathy and sensitivity		
Examiner's Global Mark	/5	
Actor / Helper's Global Mark	/5	
Total Station Mark	/30	

Learning Points:

Good history taking is essential here to include a detailed social history around the child but also the parent and extended family circle too.

Always have a high suspicion for abuse and non-accidental injury and listen carefully to pick up on hidden cues and red flags such as a changing or inconsistent history, injuries that don't fit the mechanism stated, delayed presentations and children with disabilities to name a few.

Post-operative splenectomy management includes prophylactic antibiotics to mitigate against the risks of overwhelming post-splenectomy infection.

26. Patient who wants to self-discharge / capacity assessment

Student vignette

You are the foundation year doctor in the emergency department; you have seen a 50-year-old man with a suspected new bowel malignancy that had presented with rectal bleeding. You have referred him to the surgical registrar.

The nurse has just informed you that he does not want to wait to see the surgical team and would like to self-discharge. You are asked to go and see the patient again.

After 6 minutes the examiner will stop you and ask you to summarise back your findings and ask you some direct questions.

Actor Instructions:

You are a 50-year-old man named Simon, who attended the emergency department with blood in your stools. You have been told that you have severe bleeding which may be coming from a bowel cancer and must be admitted under the surgical team for further tests and treatments. You feel otherwise well in yourself. You have been in the department for 6 hours so far. You are very agitated and want to self-discharge.

If asked why; you feel that you are too well to be admitted, you care for your elderly mother and do not want to leave her alone overnight, you feel that the surgical team are taking too long to come and see you.

Despite being offered various solutions to help with you're above concerns, you are still adamant that you wish to leave as soon as possible.

When told about the risks of ongoing bleeding, you demonstrate understanding of these risks and indicate that if things deteriorated you would seek urgent medical help again.

You ask about alternatives, accept the offer of outpatient follow up, instructions on signs of deteriorations and options to seek help.

Examiner Instructions:

The foundation year doctor in the emergency department; you have seen a 50-year-old man with a suspected new bowel malignancy who had presented with rectal bleeding. The nurse has just informed him that he does not want to wait to see the surgical team and would like to self-discharge. The candidate is asked to go and see the patient.

The scenario should be handled with subtlety and sensitivity.

After 6 minutes please bring the consultation to a close and ask the candidate the following questions for one minute:

- Can this patient safely self-discharge? Please justify your answer.

  Yes, the patient has capacity.

- What three steps are necessary before discharge?

  Inform a senior, inform the surgical team, and complete a discharge against medical advice form.

- If the patient did not have capacity, what legal framework could be used to keep the patient in hospital for investigation and treatment?

  Best interest via the Mental Capacity Act.

Please follow the mark sheet and grade appropriately.

Marksheet: Self discharge & capacity

Task:	Achieved	Not Achieved
Re-Introduces self and washes hands		
Initiates consultation with open questions		
Explores patient's concerns and reasons for wish to self-discharge		
Addresses patient's concerns and offers solutions		
Actively tries to persuade the patient to stay		
Explains plans for admission, investigations and treatment and the reasoning behind those plans		
Clearly states and explains risks of self-discharge		
Checks patient's ability to understand the information provided		
Checks patient's ability to retain information provided		
Checks patient's ability to weigh up information provided		
Check patient's ability to communicate his decision		
Offer patient alternatives management plan for follow-up and treatment		
Offers clear at home management plan including when and where to seek further help		
Maintains calm and understanding approach to the patient		
Correctly identifies that the patient has capacity		
Explains that patient can self-discharge as a patient with capacity can make an unwise decision		
States that ED seniors must be informed		
States that the surgical team must be informed		
States that relevant self-discharge forms must be completed		
Correctly identifies use of the MCA to assess and treat in best interest		
Examiner's Global Mark	/5	
Actor / Helper's Global Mark	/5	
Total Station Mark	/30	

Learning points:

You must be familiar with the capacity assessment and have an understanding of the principles behind it. Remember that a patient has the right to make an unwise decision if they have capacity. Four specific questions should be asked and documented to check that they can: understand, retain, process and weigh up and then communicate back their decision.

You should have a basic understanding of the various legal frameworks that can be used to treat a patient against their wishes such as best interest, mental capacity act and the relevant sections of the mental health act.

Pay attention to your communication skills in this station. Non-verbal skills are key. Ensure you have an open rather than defensive posture. Show active listening when the patient is expressing their concerns by nodding your head, making affirmative sounds and even repeating or summarizing their concerns back to them. Think concordance with an alternative plan rather than compliance. Offer options and create a plan that suits both you and the patient.

27. Explaining patient-controlled analgesia (PCA)

Student vignette

You are the foundation year doctor based on the surgical wards. Janet is a 55-year-old lady has been consented for an open right hemicolectomy for caecal tumour. Following this she is due to be put on a PCA for pain relief.

You have been asked by your consultant to explain what a PCA is and how it works to the patient and answer any questions they have on it.

Actor Instructions:

You are Janet, a 55-year-old lady with bowel cancer who is due to undergo an open laparotomy tomorrow. You are very concerned about the amount of pain you will be in following this procedure. The foundation year doctor on the surgical team has been asked to come and talk to you about the planned form of pain relief called a PCA or Patient Controlled Analgesia. You have not heard of this and are curious as to how it works.

You have no drug allergies and have had morphine before without any problems.

There are certain questions that you should ask over the course of the conversation:
- Can I continue to press the button constantly? What if I give myself an overdose of morphine
- I do not want to be in pain when I wake up. Can my family press the button for me while I am asleep?
- What side effects are there?
- What if it does not work? Are there any alternatives
- What happens afterwards? Do I take the PCA home?

If the explanation seems adequate to you, you should remain interested an easy to talk to – only become defensive if something is said that you do not agree with.

Examiner Instructions:

The foundation doctor has been given a scenario on pain management, they have been asked to explain what a PCA is to a patient before they have surgery tomorrow.

Please follow the mark sheet and grade appropriately.

Marksheet: Patient controlled analgesia

Task	Achieved	Not Achieved
Introduces self		
Clarifies who they are speaking to		
Clarifies patients understanding of a PCA		
Explains PCA is entirely in patient's control		
Explain that pain relief directly into a vein		
Explains that they have to press a button		
Explains that it uses morphine		
Clarifies whether any previous reaction to morphine		
Explains lockout period		
Explain that PCA is quite safe due to lockout period		
Stress that only the patient can press the button		
Explain the side effects include reduced conscious level and respiratory depression (in overdose)		
Mentions that this is the main reason no one else should push the button		
Explain that there are more options if PCA does not work		
Option 1: Increasing the dose of morphine delivered		
Option 2: Switching to a different pain killer (alfentanil for example)		
Option 3: Other forms of analgesia such as a spinal anaesthetic (Epidural)		
Explain that PCA is used for a short time and then reduced to regular analgesia		
Stresses that patient will not be going home with PCA		
Explores patients ideas, concerns and expectations		
Examiner's Global Mark	/5	
Actor/Helper Global Mark	/5	
Total	/30	

Learning Points:

IN PCA the computerized pump allows for a number of variables, including:

An initial bolus or loading dose to bring the pain under immediate control

The patient-initiated or demand dose, available to the patient at the press of a button

The delay interval or lockout, typically between six and 15 minutes, allowing the analgesic to achieve its peak effect before another dose can be administered.

The number of unsuccessful demands by patients during lockout periods is important for the physician to know.

PCAS allow a maximum volume of drug to be administered within a defined period of one, four, eight, or 24 hours, calculated to prevent an opioid overdose—regardless of how many times the PCA button gets pushED

In adults, naloxone 0.4-2mg IV can be used as a reversal agent for opioid toxicity, repeated every two minutes until full reversal.

28. Epidural Analgesia Explanation

Student vignette

A 78 year woman is due to have a Right sided total hip replacement later today. You are the foundation year doctor responsible for her care on the orthopaedic ward. The anaesthetist has been to see her and discussed having an epidural rather than a generalised anaesthetic.

Her daughter has arrived and the patient would like you to explain to her daughter how an epidural anaesthetic works and why it would be better than a general anaesthetic.

Please explain how epidural analgesia works, the broad steps involved in the procedure and its advantages and disadvantages.

After 6 minutes the examiner will stop you and ask you to summarise back your findings, and ask you some direct questions.

Actor Instructions:

You are the daughter of a 78 year old woman on the orthopaedic ward who is awaiting a right total hip replacement. Your mother and the anaesthetist have discussed anaesthetic options and decided on an epidural. You have asked your mother for details but she was vague. You have asked the junior doctor looking after your mother to explain the procedure to you.

Your main concern is to clarify what the procedure actually is. You did not have one when you delivered your child but had heard that the needle went right into the spinal column and could cut up the nerves.

You first want to know what an epidural is and how it works? Ask for confirmation that your mother will not feel anything during the procedure.

You then ask how the procedure is carried out and by whom?
You would then like to know why an epidural would be better than a general anaesthetic.
Finally you ask how long the effects of an epidural last for.

If the candidate is offering clear explanations you appear to become calmer and more reassured during the consultation.

Examiner Instructions:

The foundation doctor has been given a scenario on pain management, they have been asked to explain how epidural analgesia works, the broad steps involved in the procedure and its advantages and disadvantages.

After 6 minutes give a warning that there are 2 minutes remaining and ask the candidate the following question:

What layers will the epidural needle go through before reaching the epidural space?

Please follow the mark sheet and grade appropriately.

Marksheet: Explaining an epidural

Task:	Achieved	Not Achieved
Introduces self, washes hands and checks patient identity		
Clarifies with daughter what information she would like		
Conducts the consultation without use of excessive jargon		
Explains that an epidural is a form of regional anaesthesia		
Explains that opioid analgesics and long acting local anaesthetics are inserted into the epidural space and numb the nerves as they enter the spinal column		
Briefly describes what the epidural space is		
States that the procedure is carried out by an experienced anaesthetist in the pre-op room in theatres		
States that a fully sterile technique is used		
Describes the two positions that the procedure may be carried out in- sitting up and laying on side		
Explains that first the skin will be cleaned and anaesthetized with subcutaneous local anaesthetic		
States that a specialized needle will then be inserted carefully between the vertebra until a loss of resistance is felt		
States that once the right space is reached a small catheter (fine tube) is inserted through the needle, the needle is removed and the catheter remains in place		
Explains that the catheter will be used to inject drugs and may be attached to a patient controlled device after the procedure		
Describes the initial symptoms of warmth followed up by numbness and inability to mobilize the lower limbs		
Explains it is an alternative to general anaesthesia if GA is contra-indicated and that there is a faster recovery time, no requirement for ventilation.		

Lists potential complications such as failure, hypotension, headache, urinary retention and nausea		
Mentions rare but severe complications including bleeding, infection and nerve damage		
Explains that the effects wear off within hours of stopping the drugs but that the catheter can remain in for days post-op to aid with analgesia		
Offers opportunity to ask questions and responds appropriately		
Correctly identifies layers as skin, subcutaneous tissues, supraspinous ligament interspinous ligament, ligamentum flavum (pop often felt) and epidural space		
Examiner's Global Mark	/5	
Actor / Helper's Global Mark	/5	
Total Station Mark	/30	

Learning Points

A procedural station such as this will be testing two things. Firstly, your knowledge of the procedure. You should therefore be aware of the indications, contraindications, procedural steps, complications and basic anatomy for most common procedures.

Secondly, this station will be assessing your communication skills. You are expected to be able to elicit the information that the patient or relative wants and what their main concern is. You are also expected to be able to adapt your language and explanations to lay people with different levels of understanding.

Remember that being able to talk about a procedure does not automatically mean that you are able to consent for that procedure. GMC states that consent should be obtained by a person who is:

- a. is suitably trained and qualified
- b. has sufficient knowledge of the proposed investigation or treatment, and understands the risks involved

29. Referring a Patient to ITU (Intensive Treatment Unit)

Student vignette

You are the foundation year doctor on the general surgical team. David has been admitted under your consultant's care. He is a 57 year old gentleman who has presented with severe gallstone pancreatitis. He has severe epigastric pain radiating to his back, which is not being controlled by regular oral analgesics and PRN IV morphine.

Latest observations are:
Temperature 38.2
Heart Rate 120bpm
Blood pressure 105/65
Respiratory Rate 26 per minute

You have performed an arterial blood gas as he appeared to be becoming more breathless on air
pH 7.33   PO2 7.9
PCO2 3.5   Lac 4.3
HCO3 24

His recent blood results are:
WCC 18.6   Urea 13.2
ALT 253   LDH 420
Ca 1.9   Alb 28
Glu 7.8

After discussing the case with your senior who is in theatre, you have have been asked to contact the ITU registrar for advice and review.

The ITU on-call registrar is on the phone.

Actor Instructions

You are the ITU registrar. The foundation doctor has been asked to refer an unwell patient to you. You have had a stressful day due to a colleague calling in sick, increasing your workload so are quite blunt with the candidate.You should grudgingly accept the explanation from the candidate, especially if they stress that they are worried about the patient. They will then explain the severity of the patient's pancreatitis.

You should become more approachable if it becomes clear that the candidate has the patient's best interests at heart. You should ask the candidate why they are referring to ITU – what can ITU offer the patient that cannot be done on the ward?

Ask what treatment have they given the patient so far? Ask for recent blood tests and together create a treatment plan of IV fluids, analgelsia and strict fluid chart. Explain that ITU is almost full and there are several patients that have been referred. You should agree to go and review the patient on the ward and see whether you think they are suitable for ITU.

Examiner Instructions:

The foundation doctor has been given a scenario of severe pancreatitis, they have been asked to make a referral to the ITU Registrar. This doctor who is under a lot of pressure today due to a lack of staffing and lots of sick patients to assess and manage. They will expect a structured SBAR handover.

After 6 minutes give a warning that there are 2 minutes remaining.

Marksheet: Referral to ICU

Task	Achieved	Not Achieved
Introduction		
Clarifies who they are speaking to		
Remains polite and respectful throughout		
Purpose of referral		
Stress concern of patient safety		
Current Situation		
Background Information (blood test)		
Interprets ABG		
Explain patient has severe pancreatitis		
Mentions Glasgow Score for severity stratification		
Summarise your Assessment		
Does not make up results or investigations		
Stresses need for ITU review		
1. Invasive monitoring (Central Venous Pressure Line)		
2. Invasive monitoring (Arterial Line)		
3. Respiratory support		
Ask for Recommendation from ITU SpR		
1. 15 L oxygen		
2. Fluids, catheter hourly Urine output monitor		
Secure ITU review of patient		
Examiner's Global Mark	/5	
Actor/Helper Global Mark	/5	
Total	/30	

Learning Points:

Remember to clarify who you are speaking to and state the purpose of your call straight away. Sometimes 'headlining' with a opening statement like 'I have a patient I am worried about with probable pancreatitis' focuses the minds of both parties.

Always keep in mind that you are there representing your patient and act in their best interest to ensure they get the best quality care. Many specialist teams will be under pressure at work but you must be you patient's advocate and explain why you need that team's help.

Know the different reasons for referral to ITU. These include ventilatory support and haemofiltration and adopt a SBAR (Situation, Background, Assessment and Recommendation) approach

30. Escalating a deteriorating patient to a senior colleague

Student vignette

You are the foundation year doctor on surgical team. On a busy evening shift you are called to the ward to review a patient who the nursing staff are worried about.

The patient is a 75-year-old man who is 3 days post-Hartmann's procedure for an obstructing sigmoid tumour. His past medical history includes hypertension, poorly controlled Type 2 Diabetes and previous DVTs.

He was recovering very well and this morning and was communicating with the nursing staff normally. As the day progressed he began complaining of some abdominal pain that was relieved with morphine. However, he gradually became increasingly confused and his observations have now deteriorated. His most recent set read:

T-39.1, HR-115, BP-105/65, RR-22, Sats-93% (room air)

The nursing staff has already taken an arterial blood gas and it reads as follows:

pH: 7.25 pO2: 9.5 pCO2: 3.9 HCO3-: 14.5 BE: -4 Lactate: 4.2

You make your initial assessment and find the patient disoriented in time, place and person. He appears to be sweating and tachypnoeic. Abdominal examination reveals a peritonitic abdomen with inaudible bowel sounds on auscultation.

You decide to escalate the case to the on call surgical registrar who you know is busy in the emergency department.

Actor Instructions:

You are the surgical registrar on-call. It has been an incredibly hectic shift so far and you are still 4 hours away from finishing. You have had to take 2 emergency cases to theatre already today and are currently in the emergency department seeing a patient who is acutely unwell with Pancreatitis. You have decided i that once you have assessed and managed this patient you are going to take a break since you haven't eaten today.

You then receive a bleep from the on call foundation doctor who is requesting you come and see a patient they have assessed on the ward. Initially you are a little obstructive but If you feel the foundation doctor has conveyed the information well and highlighted the urgency then you agree to see the patient. Instruct them to commence a fast rate IV fluid infusion and to bleep the anaesthetist on-call whilst you make your way there.

Examiner instructions:

You are the foundation year doctor on surgical team. The patient is acutely unwell 3 days postoperatively with a suspected anastomotic leak.

The task of the candidate is to escalate the situation to the surgical registrar on-call for an urgent review. The registrar is very busy seeing new patients in the emergency department and will initially be obstructive about potentially coming to see the patient.

The candidate should be judged on the clarity with which they get the information across as well as how well they convince the Registrar of the urgency of the situation.

Please follow the mark sheet and grade appropriately.

Marksheet: Escalation to colleague

TASK	Achieved	Not Achieved
Introduces themselves to the Registrar		
Explains the **S**ituation: Patient name/age Summarises why they are worried		
Gives the **B**ackground: Type/date of operation Mentions the patient's PMH Patient has become increasingly confused Mentions the concerning observations Mentions the concerning results in the ABG		
Explains their **A**ssessment of the patient: Sweating Tachypnoiec General peritonitis Confusion No bowel sounds		
Gives their **R**ecommendation: Needs a urgent review from the Registrar ?anastomotic leak Asks if there is anything they can do in the meantime/suggests something		
Has an ordered, coherent structure to getting information across		
Impresses the urgency of the situation well		
Is empathic towards the registrar's situation		
Stays firm on getting the registrar to review the patient		
Delivers information confidently without much hesitation		
Examiner's global mark	/5	
Actor's global mark	/5	
Total station mark	/30	

Learning points

Practice using the **SBAR** framework for getting across information to colleagues clearly and concisely about unwell patients.

Always remember to grab the attention of a senior early by explaining WHY you are worried and the urgency of the situation.

Always put patient safety first. If a senior colleague is very busy but you still feel out of your depth you MUST flag up your concern and come to some sort of arrangement that does not jeopardise patient safety.

Chapter Three

Clinical Stations

31. Suturing under local anaesthetic

Student vignette

You are the foundation year doctor on the surgical team. A 25-year-old man named James presents with a laceration to the dorsum of his hand after cutting it against a can.

Perform an appropriate examination of the injury and close the wound using three interrupted sutures. Explain any further management.

After 6 minutes the examiner will stop you and ask you to summarise back what you have done and ask you a direct question.

Actor Instructions:

You are a 25 year old student who was playing a game of "can rip" with your friends and sustained quite a deep cut to the back of your hand. You have completely normal sensation in the hand and can move it freely. If asked about whether you have had a tetanus jab recently, answer that you "don't know what that is". You have no known allergies and no medical problems.

You are very needle phobic. Challenge the doctor at some point to whether he really has to do this to you.

Examiner Instructions:

The foundation year doctor has been asked to close a wound laceration with three simple interrupted sutures.

With two minute remaining, if the candidate has not yet advised on further management, interrupt them and prompt with the question:

'Is there anything more you would like to do or advise the patient about?'

Please follow the mark sheet and grade appropriately.

Marksheet: Suturing under local anaesthetic

Task:	Achieved	Not Achieved
Introduces self		
Clarifies the name and age of the patient		
Asks about how the injury occurred		
Asks about the patient's allergies		
Comments on the neurovascular status of the hand		
Gain consent for procedure		
Prepare the sterile field		
Cleans hands with alcohol gel		
Puts on gloves		
Cleans the area around the wound		
Administers a suitable amount (e.g. 5mls) of local anaesthetic (e.g. 1% lignocaine) around the wound site		
Specifically shows he/she is aspirating before injecting the local anaesthetic		
Tests skin to check local anaesthetic has worked		
Uses non-touch technique when manipulating the needle		
Choose correct suture type		
Applies at least two sutures across laceration with at least 3 throws		
"Wet and dry" clean after administering suture		
Applies a dressing to the site		
Asks the patient about their tetanus status & gives injection if not covered		
Consider antibiotic cover and explains that they will need to have the suture removed in 7-10 days		
Examiner's Global Mark	/5	
Actor / Helper's Global Mark	/5	
Total	/30	

Learning points

It is important to check the neurovascular status of any laceration that you see as well as potential damage to any surrounding structures. Always check the tetanus status for any patient who comes to you with a laceration.

Take time to create a good sterile field for these procedures and take especial care not to contaminate this by touching anything that is not sterile.

Known maximum dosage calculation for Lidocaine 3ml/kg and with adrenaline 6ml/kg. When choosing a suture for wound, consider properties such as non-absorbable and monofilament and the most appropriate suture size for the area of the boy effected.

32. Scrubbing

Student vignette

Your consultant requires an assistant urgently and you have been asked to scrub in to theatre. Please demonstrate your ability to scrub thoroughly, put on gloves and a surgical gown.

A cream can be applied to check your hand washing under a UV light reader.

Examiner Instructions:

The candidate has been provided with the following scenario:

Your consultant requires an assistant urgently and you have been asked to scrub in to theatre. Firstly place UV cream on candidate's hands and ask them to rub it in before scrubbing up. Test their hand washing ability by asking them to place their hands under a UV light once they have finished scrubbing, before gloving and gowning Once gowned ask them to de-gown

After 6 minutes, stop the candidate and ask them the following questions on the mark sheet.

Please follow the mark sheet and grade appropriately.

Key Points:

1. Chlorhexidine gluconate, povidone-iodine and alcohol are the commonly used antiseptics. Keep practising on scrubbing and closed glove technique

2. Disinfection only reduces the number of viable microorganisms. Sterilization kills all viable microorganisms.

3. Chlorhexidine based antiseptic preparations are more effective in reducing bacterial concentration and longer lasting effect than iodine preparations.

Marksheet: Scrubbing

Task:	Achieved	Not Achieved
Gather Equipment		
Introduction to Theatre Team		
Gather equipment		
Offer to change into theatre scrubs, change into theatre shoes		
Wear theatre cap		
Wear theatre mask to cover nose and mouth fully		
Expose hands and forearms to elbows		
Wash hands,		
Open gown and gloves in a sterile manner		
Perform pre-scrub wash for one minute, fingers/arms/elbows		
Nailbrush Use and Keep elbows below your hands so that the dirty water runs away		
Perform three scrub cleaning technique: Fingers/Palms/ Arms (UV Cream)		
Examine hands under UV Light		
Dry hands with sterile paper towels		
Put Gown on, ensuring fingers are not exposed		
Closed gloving sterile technique		
Keep hands above elbows		
Hand your assistant the belt tie and turn around to then secure waist belt		
De-gown and Wash hands		
Examples of commonly used antiseptics		
Define disinfection and sterilization		
Examiner's Global Mark	/5	
Actor / Helper's Global Mark	/5	
Total Station Mark	/30	

Learning Points:

Good hand hygiene is important throughout the clinical environment. Make sure you know a methodical technique to ensure all areas are cleaned be it with either soap and water or alcohol gel.

'Scrubbing in' formally will reduces the risk of infection and thus significantly improves patient outcomes. This is a skill that needs to be equally well by a medical student or consultant and should be taken very seriously and always performed to the highest standard.

Gowning up will always require another person to aide you. Do not try and cut corners and do things yourself as this will lead to error and contamination.

33. ATLS – C- Spine Immobilization and Rigid Collar Measurement

Student vignette

You are a foundation doctor in the emergency department. A cyclist has been brought in after a collision. He is currently lying on a spinal board but his C-Spine has not been immobilised and he is not wearing a collar.

You have been asked to do this with the assistance of an actor, who will play the role of a medical student. You will need to instruct the actor as to their role and requirements. You can presume the cyclist has no other injuries.

Actor Instructions

You are a medical student on the first day of your emergency department placement who offers assistance to the foundation doctor in the immobilization of the c-spine.

You will only assist following instructions from the candidate. You are not to direct the candidate in any way.

Examiner Instructions

This station is testing whether the candidate can safely and effectively immobilize the c-spine and measure a rigid collar. They have been instructed that they have the assistance of a medical student who is new to the ED who has no trauma training. The candidate must instruct the assistant. The actor will follow instructions from the candidate only.

Please follow the mark sheet and grade appropriately.

Marksheet: Applying a Cervical spine collar

Task:	Achieved	Not Achieved
Introduces self		
Clarifies the name of patient		
Explains procedure to patient		
Explains procedure to assistant		
Reassures patient		
Gathers equipment: Spinal board (patient positioned on) Rigid neck collar Supportive blocks Tape		
Places neck in neutral position (this may be actively or passively – stops if pain worsens)		
Instructs assistant to immobilise in the neutral position. Either done by passing hands either side of the head to the trapezius muscles or thumbs anteriorly and fingers posteriorly clamping the head in between.		
Determine collar size (5 marks) Using fingers widths, measure the vertical distance from the top of the shoulder to an imaginary line at the base of the chin Then find the appropriately sized collar Align the bottom of the collar to the finger widths of the patient using the marker stud Insert strap end of collar under neck Secure collar using velcro strap		
Supportive blocks to be applied either side of the head and actor instructed to remove hands from immobilising neck.		
Tape is to be used across the chin and across the forehead: Right side of backboard to the inferior right edge of block across chin, inferior edge of left block onto backboard. Repeat above across patient's forehead and the superior aspects of the block 2 marks		
Explains what they are doing throughout to the patient		

Examiner's Global Mark	/5	
Actor / Helper's Global Mark	/5	
Total Station Mark	/30	

Learning Points

Pre hospital patients will be packaged with a spinal board and c spine collar but on arrival to the ED a rapid assessment should be made utilising the NICE or canadian c spine neck imaging rules to stratify the investigations needed or to be able to remove the collar.

Prolonged immobilization on a long spinal board and use of a cervical collar are associated with notable morbidity most commonly secondary to cutaneous pressure necrosis.

Rigid cervical collars are used to aid C-spine immobilization as they limit flexion and extension, lateral bending and rotation and must only be used with in-line or mechanical immobilisation.

34. Management of airway including adjuncts

Student vignette

You are the foundation year doctor attached to the on-call surgical team. A car crash has occurred nearby and several trauma calls have arrived in the hospital at the same time. Your registrar has asked you to begin a primary survey on John, who has come in unconscious while he deals with another trauma.

During this station you will be asked to demonstrate airway management on a manikin and answer questions posed by the examiner.

Actor Instructions:

For this station you will need a manikin and airway adjuncts for the candidate to demonstrate their technique.

A car crash has occurred nearby and several trauma calls have arrived in the hospital at the same time. The registrar has asked the candidate to begin a primary survey on John, who has come in unconscious while he deals with another trauma.

During this station they will be asked to demonstrate airway management on a manikin and answer questions posed by the examiner.

The candidate should check responsiveness of the patient whilst introducing himself or herself to the patient. At this point state 'the patient is not responding'.

The candidate should then look, listen and feel for breath sounds for 10 seconds. State that they can see the chest rising and falling, and they can hear breath sounds, which sound like snoring. The candidate should then perform an airway manoeuvre. This should be a jaw thrust, as the c spine has not been cleared. If the candidate performs a jaw thrust ask them 'why did you not use the head tilt chin lift technique?' Answer should be that the C spine has not been cleared.

The candidate should then move on to using an airway adjunct. They should have a choice of several different sizes of oropharyngeal airways and nasopharyngeal airways. They should choose an oropharyngeal airway and measure it appropriately. They should then insert it into the manikin. Ask 'why did you not choose the nasopharyngeal airway?' Answer should be the risk of a skull base fracture.

Tell the candidate that the patient is tolerating the airway and there are no more added breath sounds. Ask the candidate 'what would you do next?'

Stop the scenario and remove the oropharyngeal airway. Ask the candidate to demonstrate the airway manoeuvre and adjunct that they did not use previously.

Examiner Instructions:

For this station you will need a CPR manikin and airway adjuncts for the candidate to demonstrate their technique with.

Guide the student through the scenario as the actor with manikin

Please follow the mark sheet and grade appropriately.

Marksheet: Airway adjuncts

Task	Achieved	Not Achieved
Wash hands		
Introduces self		
Checks response		
Call for help		
Look, listen and feel for breath sounds		
Identifies need for airway manoeuvre		
Chooses to perform jaw thrust		
Demonstrates jaw thrust adequately		
Explains need for c spine clearance before head tilt chin lift can be considered		
Identifies the need for airway adjunct		
Chooses oropharyngeal airway		
Sizes oropharyngeal airway correctly		
Inserts airway in correct fashion		
Applies oxygen on patient		
Ensures resolution of added breath sounds		
Explains danger of nasopharyngeal tube in trauma with regards to skull base fracture		
Describes escalation to BVM, iGel and intubation if apnoeic		
Mentions would go on to assess and manage breathing and circulation		
Mentions need for anaesthetic input early on		
Demonstrates head tilt chin lift adequately		
Demonstrates nasopharyngeal airway insertion adequately		
Examiner's Global Mark	/5	
Actor/Helper Global Mark	/5	
Total	/30	

Learning Points:

Knowing how to properly insert airway adjuncts is a simple yet important skill that can buy time before a definitive airway is placed. Practice sizing and placing both oropharyngeal and nasopharyngeal airways.

If an airway adjunct is tolerated it suggests a GCS of 8 or less. This requires urgent ITU assessment for a definitively airway. Good basic airway management can save lives though so there must be no delay waiting for seniors.

It is important not to do further harm in a trauma. If c spine has not been cleared then jaw thrust is the airway manoeuvre of choice. This will require more personnel with one person to maintain the jaw thrust and another to place the oropharyngeal airway.

35. Surgical Chest Drain insertion

Student vignette

You are a foundation doctor working in the Emergency Department. A 71-year-old man was brought in an hour ago as a trauma call. He was a restrained driver of a car who crashed into a tree at 45 mph. He has had a full primary and secondary survey and has just come back from a CT scan to the resuscitation department. The CT shows the only injury sustained is a right-sided pneumothorax and you have just reviewed these images yourself. The Emergency Department consultant has said he'll supervise and assist you putting in your first surgical chest drain.

Before starting the procedure tell the consultant what equipment you will need, and how you wish to prepare the patient. Then turn to the patient and insert the chest drain.

Actor's Instructions:

You are a 71-year-old male named Ahmed, you are very stoical and are in sound mind after crashing your car. You understand that you are going to need a chest drain for a pneumothorax as you are a retired GP. You take no regular medication and have no allergies.

Ask the candidate what painkillers they are going to give you before they start.

Examiner's instructions:

The candidate has seen a 71-year-old man was brought in an hour ago as a trauma call. He was a restrained driver of a car who crashed into a tree at 45 mph. He had a full primary and secondary survey; a CT scan has confirmed the only injury sustained is a right-sided pneumothorax. The Emergency Department consultant has said he'll supervise and assist the foundation doctor putting in their first surgical chest drain.

The purpose of this task is to assess the knowledge required to insert a surgical chest drain:

- The candidate knows the required equipment
- The candidate knows how best to prepare the patient
- The candidate knows the steps to safely insert a chest drain

Assist the candidate by organising their equipment and preparing the sterile field. Before the candidate makes an incision ask them what are the anatomical borders of the safe triangle.

Marksheet: Chest drain insertion

Task:	Achieved	Not Achieved
Introduces self, clarifies the name and age of the patient		
Gets verbal consent		
Prepares equipment: needle, syringe, local anaesthetic, sterile wound pack, skin prep, sterile gloves, scalpel, Roberts or similar instrument, 28-32F chest drain and under water collecting bottle.		
Asks about the patient's allergies		
Puts patient into a suitable position eg. 45° on a bed with their right hand behind their head		
Discusses the need for patient monitoring during the procedure – with or without sedation.		
Cleans hands and puts on gloves		
Keeps the sterile field		
Anatomically defines the safe triangle		
Cleans the skin prior to local anaesthetic		
Safely injects local anaesthetic (e.g. 1% lignocaine) first to the skin, then the intercostal muscles and down to the pleura		
Tests skin to check local anaesthetic has worked		
Makes an incision above an appropriate rib		
Bluntly dissects down to and through the pleura		
Finger sweep inside chest		
Introduces the drain a suitable distance atraumatically using Roberts		
Attaches drain to collecting system		
Checks that the drain is "swinging"		
Fixes (eg sutures) drain in place appropriately		
Gets a CXR to check position of the drain		
Examiner's Global Mark	/5	
Actor / Helper's Global Mark	/5	
Total Station Mark	/30	

Learning points:

It is important to appreciate the difference between a simple pneumothorax, which needs draining within hours and a tension pneumothorax with is an emergency and needs draining within minutes.

Careful consideration of the anatomical landmarks will reduce the risk of iatrogenic injury to surrounding structure. Beware of the neurovascular bundle below each rib.

This is not a routine procedure that a foundation doctor would be expected to perform. it is however essential to know the indications for thoracocentesis and chest drain insertion and also good practice to know the equipment and methodology as you may well assist your senior in these procedures.

36. Femoral arterial blood Sampling

Student vignette

You are the foundation year doctor, part of the on call medical resuscitation team. You receive a peri-arrest call to attend.

On arrival you find a 60-year-old patient with deteriorating observations and poorly perfused peripheries. The registrar leading the team instructs you to perform a femoral arterial stab.

Gather the appropriate equipment for this task and simulate the method of performing this procedure on a manikin. Please explain your steps whilst going along.

Examiner Instructions:

The foundation year doctor has been asked to perform a femoral arterial sample.

The purpose of this task is to assess the following:

- Correct technique for performing femoral arterial stab
- Appropriate identification of anatomy

Please follow the mark sheet and grade appropriately.

Marksheet: Femoral Stab

TASK	Achieved	Not Achieved
Introduces self and confirms correct patient		
Verbally consents the patient		
Gathers equipment of items: Chloroprep, Syringe, Needle, blood bottles, Gauze + tape		
Washes hands		
Applies gloves		
Describes exposing the patient adequately		
Mentions feeling for the landmarks: ASIS, Pubic symphysis		
Describes finding the femoral artery at the mid-inguinal point (midway between the 2 landmarks)		
Comment on the Femoral sheath content		
Cleans Skin with chlorprep		
Describes inserting the needle at a right angle to the skin		
Pulls back on syringe ensuring no pulsation of blood suggesting an arterial stab		
Applies pressure to the area with gauze once the sample is taken		
Tapes down the gauze after applying pressure		
Puts the sample in the blood bottles		
Labels the bottles at bedside		
Dispose of sharps safely		
Removes gloves and washes hands post-procedure		
Completes blood forms with date, time, signature		
Documents procedure and bloods taken in notes		
Examiner's global mark	/5	
Actor/Helper's global mark	/5	
Total station mark	/30	

Learning points

Remember that the mid-inguinal point is the midpoint of a straight line drawn from the tip of the Anterior Superior Iliac Spine to the pubic symphysis.

Remember the order of the neurovascular bundle in the femoral triangle Lateral to medial: NAVY, boundaries of femoral canal and femoral triangle

Always remember to wash your hands before AND AFTER patient contact. Wearing gloves is not an excuse to cut corners on handwashing.

37. Ankle Brachial Pressure Index

Student vignette

You have been asked to see a 72-year-old woman who has presented to the vascular clinic complaining of pain in her calves on walking.

You are the foundation doctor on the Vascular Team and have been asked to perform an ankle brachial pressure index and report your results to the vascular team.

Actor Instructions

You are a 72-year-old lady, called Sarah, who has been referred to the vascular team from your GP with pain in the back of your calves. This has been going on for four months and is brought on by walking. You notice that the pain eases the moment you stop.

You are a type 2 diabetic and have had a heart stent in the past for heart disease. You have not had any heart attacks of strokes however. You have no allergies and take metformin and gliclazide for your diabetes and simvastatin, ramipril and bisoprolol for you heart. You are a non- smoker.

The foundation doctor has been asked by the team to perform an ABPI before you see the consultant.

Examiner's Instructions

A 72-year-old female has presented to the vascular clinic complaining of pain in her calves on walking. The foundation doctor on the vascular team has been asked to perform an ankle brachial pressure index (ABPI) and report their results to the rest of the vascular team.

Please observe the candidate perform an ABPI and assess them according to the mark scheme.

Marksheet: ABPI

Task	Achieved	Not Achieved
Introduces self, washes hands and checks patient identity		
Lays patient supine and adequately exposes patient		
Ensures that leg have been rested for >20mins		
Select appropriate sized BP cuff and places around arm		
Palpate brachial artery and applied Ultrasound Gel		
Use Doppler probe to locate brachial pulse and inflate cuff till Doppler disappears, deflates and records pressure at which signal returns		
Cleans gel and offers to repeat process for other arm		
States would use higher of 2 brachial systolic readings to calculi ABPI		
Select appropriate sized BP cuff and places above the malleoli		
Locate Dorsalis Pedis (DP) pulse by palpation or applied Ultrasound gel and uses Doppler		
Continue as for the brachial pulse and records DP pressure		
Repeats for Posterior Tibial (PT) pulse and records PT pulse pressure		
Uses the higher of the two readings when calculating ABPIs for ankle		
Offers to repeat for other leg		
Cleans ultrasounds gel from skin and restores patient's modesty		
Washes hands		
Calculates and documents ABPI's in patient notes		
Presentation of findings with interpretation of results		
Awareness of patients needs through examination		
Professionalism		
Examiner's Global Mark	/5	
Actor / Helper's Global Mark	/5	
Total Station Mark	/30	

Learning Points

Ensure patient is lying flat before you start and that the legs aren't hanging over the bed.

This basic technique compares the 'best' estimate of non-invasive measured central systolic blood pressure, that is the highest of the two brachial systolic pressures as measured by Doppler, with the highest pressure recorded from the vessels at the ankle

The cut off for ABPI are:
>0.9-1.2- normal
>
> <0.9->0.5- mild to moderate- patient may be asymptomatic or have intermittent claudication
>
> <0.5- Critical limb ischaemic- Patient may complain of rest pain and are put at increased risk of non- healing ulcer of gangrene

38. Male catheterisation

Student vignette

You have been asked to see a 72-year-old male, who has not been able to pass urine for the last 8 hours and is complaining of severe abdominal pain. Your team suspect that he is in urinary retention.

You are the foundation doctor on the Urology team and have been asked to take a focused history, perform a brief examination and then catheterise the patient.

After 6 minutes the examiner will stop you and ask you to summarise back your findings and your management plan.

Actor Instructions

You are a 72-year-old man, named Colin, who has come in complaining of severe lower abdominal pain that comes in waves. You feel an urge to pass urine but have not been able to do so for the last 8 hours. You have had problems with your "waterworks" for the last 3-4 months, namely getting up 4-5 times a night to pass urine. In addition when you go to the toilet you feel that you have to go urgently and can't wait, you have had the embarrassing episode of wetting your trousers once or twice in the last month.

When you go you notice that it takes you a little while to get started and the urine seems to just trickle out rather than form a strong stream. You have noticed that at the end of the episode you are still passing small amounts of urine. On average a day you go to the toilet every couple of hours.

You are otherwise well but have had a heart attack in the past when you were 64 and have a history of a coronary artery bypass graft carried out 4 years ago. You are a type 2 diabetic who controls their diabetes with metformin and gliclazide. You also have some heart medication, the names of which you are unsure about. You have a family history of heart disease and lung cancer.

You have spoken to your GP 1 month ago about your urinary problem and he has started you on two medications for your prostate. Tamsulosin and Finasteride, so far these have helped a little. You are waiting for an appointment with the urology team.

On examination you are exquisitely tender in your lower abdomen and have noticed a large lump forming. The nurses have completed a "bladder scan" which shows 820mls in your bladder.

Examiner Instructions

A 72-year-old male has presented to the emergency department complaining that he has not been able to pass urine in 8 hours despite wanting to go and is now complaining of severe abdominal pain.

The foundation doctor on the Urology Team has been asked to catheterise the patient as the team suspect urinary retention and take focused history and examination and then summarise the findings back to the team.

After 6 minutes stop the candidate and ask them to please summarise their findings and management plan.

Marksheet: catheterisation

Task	Achieved	Not Achieved
Introduces self & washes hands		
Offers chaperone		
Examination of abdomen in concise manner		
Selects 16Fr catheter for insertion		
Positions patient on his back with legs slight apart and lying flat		
Open's catheter pack using aseptic technique		
Washes and dries hands and then puts on sterile gloves		
Drapes the patient and places a collecting vessel in between the legs		
Retracts foreskin		
Holds penis with sterile swab and cleans penis and around meatus ensuring only 1 swipe is used per swab		
Inserts anaesthetic gel and waits for effect		
Holds penis vertically with one hand and holds catheter tip by its sleeve		
Advances catheter into urethra ensuring it is advanced in the neck		
Waits until urine is flowing		
Inflates balloon using 10mls of sterile water (does not do so until urine is flowing)		
Attaches catheter bag		
Replaces foreskin		
Dispose of gloves and washes hand. Clears away using appropriate		
Measures residual in catheter bag		
Documents appropriately in the notes		
Examiner's Global Mark /5		
Actor / Helper's Global Mark /5		
Total Station Mark /30		

Learning Points

Simple strategies can go a long way to ensuring a successful catheterisation. Preparation of the correct equipment in particular the catheter size is vital. Ensuring that the penis is orientated vertical before insertion. This ensures that the urethra is straightened.

Once the catheter has been passed wait to inflate the catheter balloon urine is freely draining. If urine is not draining the catheter may still be in the urethra and inflation of balloon may cause urethral damage.

It is essential to ensure that the foreskin if present is replaced as a retracted foreskin significantly increases risk of paraphimosis. This should be documented in the notes.

39. Female Catheterisation

Student vignette

You are the foundation doctor attached to the Urology Team. A 47-year-old lady has come to the emergency department with a blocked catheter. You have been asked by the Urology Team to see her and change her catheter.

Actor Instructions

You are 47-year-old woman, named Bridget, who has a background of multiple sclerosis. As a result you have a long-term catheter because you can no longer control your bladder. You have your catheter changed regularly by the district nurse, however you have noticed that your catheter has not been draining.

You also noticed that your urine has become cloudier and smellier over the last few days and are worried that you may have picked up an infection. As a result, you called an ambulance to go to the Emergency Department so you can get checked over by a doctor.

Examiner Instructions

A 47-year-old lady has presented to the Emergency Department with a blocked catheter. The foundation doctor has been asked by the Urology Team to see her and change her catheter if necessary.

Please observe the candidate perform a female catheterisation and assess them according to the mark scheme.

Marksheet: Female catheterisation

Task	Achieved	Not Achieved
Introduces self & washes hands		
Offers chaperone		
Examination of abdomen in concise manner		
Selects appropriate size catheter for insertion (12-14Fr)		
Positions patient on her back with ankles together and knees falling apart to the side		
Exposes patient adequately and maintains privacy		
Open's catheter pack using aseptic technique		
Aseptic set's up all equipment		
Washes and dries hands and then puts on sterile gloves		
Drapes the patient and places a collecting vessel		
Parts labia with one hand and cleans urethra using single downward wipe		
Inserts anaesthetic gel and waits for effect.		
Parts labia with one hand and holds catheter tip by its sleeve in the other.		
Advances catheter into urethra		
Waits until urine is flowing		
Inflates balloon using 10mls of sterile water (does not do so until urine is flowing)		
Maintains sterility at all times		
Attaches catheter bag		
Dispose of gloves and washes hands. Clears away equipment using appropriate technique		
Measures residual in catheter bag		
Examiner's Global Mark /5		
Actor / Helper's Global Mark /5		
Total Station Mark /30		

Learning Points

Female catheterisation differs from male catheterisation as because the urethra is much shorter, the catheter does not need to be advanced as far.

Women are at increased risk of urinary tract infection as their urethra are shorter and they lack the "spiral mechanism" present in men during micturition which serves to clean the external urethral meatus.

When performing intimate examinations, it is essential that you have a chaperone with you to safeguard both yourself and the patient. Documenting this clearly in the notes.

40. Insertion of a Nasogastric Tube

Student vignette

You are the foundation doctor on a General Surgery team. During the morning ward round your consultant asks you to insert a nasogastric tube for Tammy to drain her stomach as she has small bowel obstruction and has been vomiting. One of the ward nurses will assist you.

Please explain your steps to the examiner as you perform the procedure.

Actor Instructions

You are Tammy a 63-year-old female who has been admitted to the surgical ward after coming into the emergency department for vomiting.

You have been told you have a bowel obstruction and will need a nasogastric tube inserted as part of your management.

Examiner's instructions:

The purpose of this task is to assess the following:

- Correct technique for insertion of a nasogastric tube
- Can identify misplacement of the tube

When the candidate has inserted the tube ask them "which investigation would you use to check the position?"

Show the candidate the CXR below and ask them to comment on its position. Please follow the mark sheet and grade appropriately.

Marksheet: NG Tube placement

TASK	Achieved	Not Achieved
Introduces self to patient		
Explains the procedure to the patient		
Gains verbal consent		
Washes hands and puts on gloves		
Correctly selects the wider bore tube for aspiration		
Positions the patient sitting up in bed with their head against a pillow		
Measures the approximate length from the patient's nose to their stomach and records the distance		
Uses appropriate adjuncts to assist placement of the tube e.g. lubrication and asking the patient to swallow water		
Insert the tube into a patent nostril aiming along the floor of the nose		
Insert the tube so that the natural curvature of the tube is along the floor of the nose		
When the tube enters the oropharynx rotate 180° to discourage the tube entering the mouth		
Advance the tube into the oesophagus and stomach whilst asking the patient to swallow.		
Measures an appropriate distance 50-60cm		
Attaches a drainage bag to the tube		
Secures the tube in place with tape to the nose		
Checks position in stomach by using litmus paper to test the pH of the aspirate		
Asks to check position of the tube with CXR		
Notes the incorrect position of the tube		
Suggests immediate removal of the tube		
Checks that the patient is ok after insertion		
Examiner's global mark	/5	
Actor/Helper's global mark	/5	
Total station mark	/30	

Ask the candidate to identify the position of the NGT on this CXR.

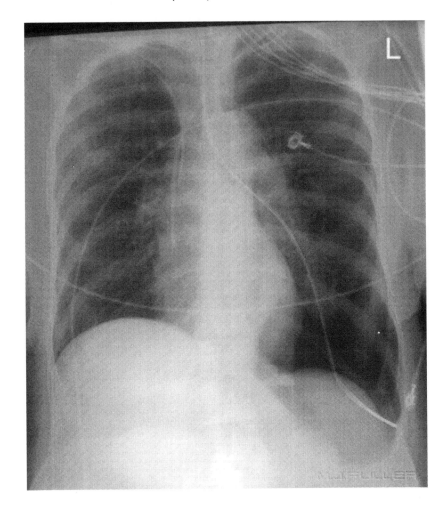

Learning points

If tube insertion fails at the level of the nose try the other nostril. Never force the tube as if there is an obstruction such as a polyp it could bleed profusely if it is traumatised.

Large bore nasogastric tubes, for example size 16 or 12 are appropriate for aspiration, finer bore tubes, for example 9 are more appropriate for NG feeding.

Feeding a patient down a misplaced nasal tube into the lungs is a "never event" and safety steps should be employed to ensure it never happens. A CXR should be performed every time before a tube is used to feed.

41. Abdominal Radiograph Interpretation

Student vignette

You are the foundation year doctor in general surgery. A 72-year-old female patient with a background of relapsing remitting multiple sclerosis presents to the acute surgical take. She describes severe generalised abdominal pain. You request an abdominal radiograph to investigate for an underlying cause. You are now asked by the consultant on the post take ward round to describe the abdominal radiograph in a systematic manner, assemble a differential diagnosis and management plan for this patient.

Abdominal plain radiograph examples for Interpretation:

Example one:

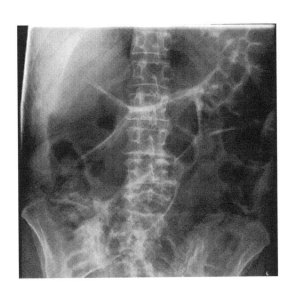

Example two:

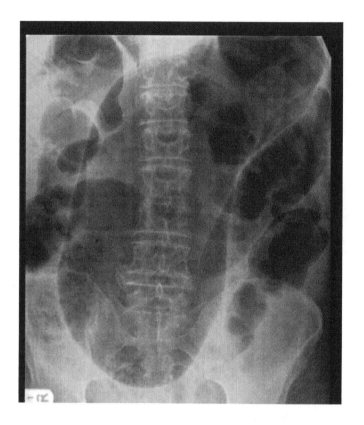

Example three:

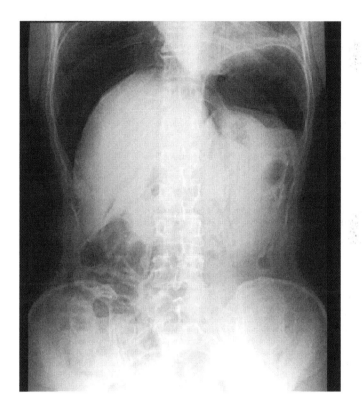

Example four:

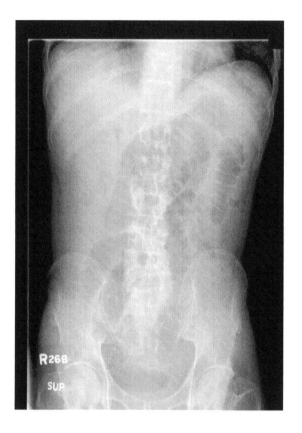

Examiner Instructions:

The candidate will be required to describe the plain abdominal radiograph presented to them (one of four examples).

The candidate will be allowed a pen and paper to scribe notations to aid in the presentation of their findings. No comments from the examiner will be provided during this assessment.

At six minutes the candidate should summarise their findings, presenting the abdominal x ray in an informed and logical and systematic manner. It must be appreciated by the examiner that there are different techniques in presenting plain radiographs, as long as the key points are reviewed, the candidate will score.

Please follow the mark sheet and grade appropriately.

Task:	Achieved	Not Achieved
Introduces self & washes hands		
Clarifies whom they are speaking to.		
Comment on date of radiograph		
Correct Patient details (DOB & Hospital No)		
Projection of image – Anterior –Posterior		
Comments on adequacy of the image		
Comments on the rotation		
Comments on the penetration		
Comment on bowel gas pattern		
Bowel 3cm, 6 cm, 9 cm – normal anatomical width of small bowel, large bowel and caecum.		
Comment on Small bowel identified (i.e. Valvulae conniventes described if present)		
Comment on Large bowel identified (i.e.haustra described if present)		
Comment on pathology such as volvulus		
Comment on faecal loading		
Other organs: Soft tissue shadows – liver, spleen, kidneys, gall bladder, psoas shadow.		
Bone: The lower ribs, lumbar vertebrae, sacrum, coccyx, pelvic bones		
Comment on any calcification and artifact		
Summarize findings		
Provide differential diagnosis and further investigations		
Comment on your management plan for this patient		
Examiner's Global Mark	/5	
Actor / Helper's Global Mark	/5	
Total Station Mark	/30	

Learning Points

Example one demonstrates large bowel obstruction. The most common aetiology of large bowel obstructions are colorectal cancer and diverticular strictures. Dilatation of the caecum >9cm is considered abnormal.

Example two demonstrates sigmoid volvulus. The sigmoid colon is more prone to twisting than other segments of the large bowel because it is 'mobile' on its own mesentery. Treatment is decompression of the volvulus with rigid/flexible sigmoidoscopy.

Example four demonstrates small bowel obstruction. Plain radiograph will demonstrate centrally located multiple dilated loops of gas filled bowel. The valvulae conniventes are visible. This confirms small bowel involvement.

42. Chest Radiograph Interpretation

Student vignette

You are the foundation year doctor in general surgery. A 72-year-old presents with severe generalised abdominal pain with shortness of breath on exertion. You request an erect chest radiograph to investigate for an underlying cause.

You are now asked by the consultant on the post take ward round to describe the chest radiograph in a systematic manner, assemble a differential diagnosis and management plan for this patient.

Chest plain radiograph examples for Interpretation

1. *Example of air under diaphragm*

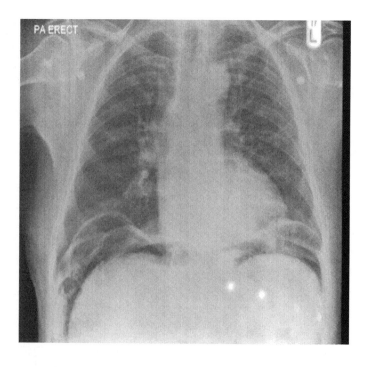

2. *Example left rib fractures with surgical chest drain*

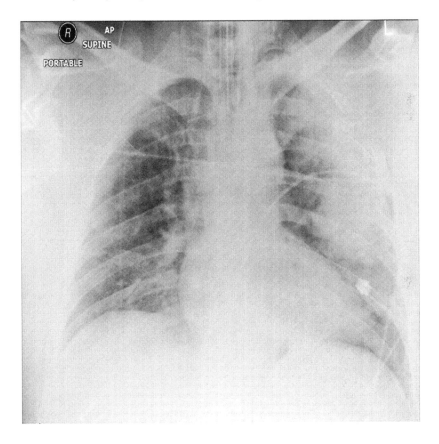

3. *Example of left pneumothorax, signs of early tension*

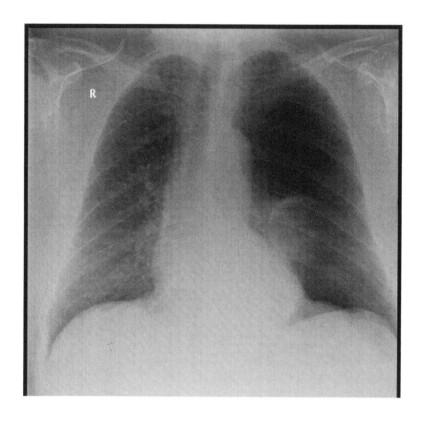

4. *Example of Aortic injury*

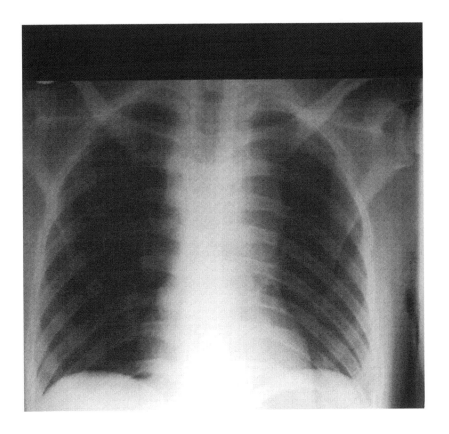

Examiner Instructions:

The candidate will be required to describe the plain chest radiograph presented to them (one of four examples).

The candidate will be allowed a pen and paper to scribe notations to aid in the presentation of their findings. No comments from the examiner will be provided during this assessment.

At six minutes the candidate should summarise their findings, presenting the abdominal x ray in an informed and logical and systematic manner. It must be appreciated by the examiner that there are different techniques in presenting plain radiographs, as long as the key points are reviewed, the candidate will score. Please follow the mark sheet and grade appropriately.

Marksheet: CXR interpretation

Task	Achieved	Not Achieved
Introduces self and washes hands		
Clarifies whom they are speaking to		
Comment on date of radiograph		
Correct Patient Details (D.O.B. & Hospital No:)		
Projection of image – Anterior-Posterior		
Quality of Image – Adequacy		
Rotation		
Penetration		
Airway – Tracheal Deviation		
Breathing – Lung Fields, Pneumothorax, Lobar Collapse		
Hilar Lymphadenopathy		
Circulation – Heart Size, Heart Position		
Great vessels, Mediastinal Width <8cm on PA		
Diaphragm – Position and Shape, Costo-phrenic angles		
Air below diaphragm		
Bones, Artefacts		
Soft Tissues- Looking for masses, subcutaneous, calcification of aorta		
Summarize Findings		
Provides differential diagnosis and further investigations		
Comment on a management plan for the radiograph		
Examiner's Global Mark	/ 5	
Actor /Helper's Global Mark	/ 5	
Total Station Mark	/ 30	

Learning Points

Patient details are the most simple and important point. Always start with checking the film bears the patient's name, date of birth and hospital number and is the image taken today. With the advent of digital image banks it is very easy to open the wrong image.

Example one is an example of pneumoperitoneum, most likely due to a visceral perforation that is a surgical emergency. Example two shows rib fractures and a surgical drain placed likely due to trauma. Such a patient should be managed in an ATLS trauma call manner.

Being able to identify CXR findings is essential as a junior doctor but knowing the initial management of each of these diagnoses is even more important. Learning the BTS guidelines for management for pneumothorax treatment for example is a core piece of knowledge for doctors.

Chapter Four
Examination Stations

43. Examination of an Abdominal Stoma

Student vignette

You are the foundation year doctor on the surgical team. Smitha is a 72-year-old lady who has undergone abdominal surgery and has a stoma.

Your consultant asks you to examine the patient's stoma on the ward round.

Actor Instructions:

You are Smitha, a 72-year-old lady, who underwent an emergency Hartmanns procedure for a perforation secondary to severe diverticular disease. You have been left with an end colostomy.

Please do not give any information other than explaining you are not in pain if asked.

Examiner Instructions:

The foundation year doctor has been asked to perform a stoma examination on a 72 year-old lady who has undergone abdominal surgery and has an end colostomy stoma.

After 6 minutes stop the candidate and ask them to 'please summarise your findings, including a differential diagnosis and immediate management plan' for 2 minutes.

Please follow the mark sheet and grade appropriately.

Marksheet: Examination of an Abdominal Stoma

Task	Achieved	Not Achieved
Wash Hands, Introduction and Consent		
Requests a chaperone		
Expose & Position Patient		
General Inspection hands, pulse, eyes, mouth		
Remove stoma bag		
Comment on scars and colour of stoma		
Site of stoma		
Surrounding skin		
Comment on stoma contents and output		
No: Lumens and Shape (Spout or flushed)		
Comment on whether there is a parastomal hernia, prolapse, retraction		
Ask if patient is in pain before palpation		
Digital stoma examination		
Comment on patency or stenosis features		
Trans illuminate, assess stoma mucosa		
Reattach stoma bag		
Thank patient and wash hands		
Present findings		
Name the type of stoma and why patient likely required this operation		
How are stomas classified?		
Examiner's Global Mark	/5	
Actor / Helper's Global Mark	/5	
Total Station Mark	/30	

Learning Points:

To complete stoma examination always mention you will like to do a full abdominal examination, inspect the perineum for scars and patency of anus as well as evaluating the stoma position while standing and sitting

Stomas are classified as Loop VS End, Temporary VS Permanent and anatomical site

Always divided stoma complications into early (ischemia, obstruction, retraction) and late (stenosis, fistula formation, parastomal hernia)

44. Examination of an Acute Abdomen

Student vignette

You are an foundation year doctor working in General Surgery. You receive a call from your Registrar, who is in theatre, asking you to examine the abdomen of Reuben who is a 50 year old man in the Surgical Admissions Unit. The patient was seen earlier in the day by their GP and referred directly to the surgical team with an acute abdomen. He has central severe pain, which started suddenly four hours ago.

Explain to the examiner what you are doing as you conduct your abdominal examination. The examiner will provide you with the clinical findings that you request.

Actor Instructions:

You are a 50-year-old man who has had severe upper abdominal pain for the last 4 hours. You are breathing quite fast and are dehydrated and thirsty. You have pain when your abdomen is pushed all over your abdomen. The pain makes you contract your abdominal muscles. The worst pain is in the upper abdomen.

Follow the instructions of the doctor examining you.

Examiner Instructions:

The foundation year doctor has been asked to perform an abdominal examination on a 50 year old man who has presented with acute generalized abdominal pain

You must relay the below information to the candidate when it is appropriate. After 6 minutes, stop the candidate and ask him what further examinations he would like to perform, what investigations he would like, and ask for three possible diagnoses.

	Clinical findings
End of the bed	Looks generally unwell
Hands and nails	Cool and clammy, normal nails
Pulse	110 beats per minute
Examines the face	Dry mucus membranes Sunken eyes Normal conjunctiva Normal skin colour
Inspects abdomen	Mildly distended abdomen Open Appendicectomy Scar
Palpates abdomen for tenderness	Rigid abdomen – epigastric area most tender. Guarding in upper abdomen.
Palpates abdomen for masses	No masses and no abnormal pulsations
Palpates abdomen for Liver, Spleen and Kidneys	Normal
Percusses abdomen	Normal percussion but results in pain in the upper abdomen
Auscultates abdomen	Absent bowel sounds
Examines hernial orifices	No hernias present

The observations are:
Heat Rate – 110bpm, Respiratory Rate – 30bpm, Blood Pressure 100/70, Temperature 38.5°C, Oxygen Saturations 96% on Air

Please follow the mark sheet and grade appropriately.

Marksheet: Examination of the acute abdomen

Task:	Achieved	Not Achieved
Washes their hands, introduces themselves and obtains consent for the examination		
Examines patient from the end of the bed		
Checks hands and nails		
Pulse		
Examines the face / sclera for jaundice		
Examines the conjunctiva for pallor		
Examines the mucus membranes for hydration		
Exposes the abdomen and positions the patient flat then inspects for distension, scars and abnormal movements		
Palpates abdomen methodically in 9 sections		
Palpates abdomen for masses		
Palpates abdomen for Liver, Spleen and ballots the Kidneys		
Percusses abdomen		
Auscultates abdomen (bruits and bowel sounds)		
Examines hernial orifices		
Suggests DRE and examination of the external genitalia to complete the examination		
Thank patient and wash hands		
Summarize findings		
Asks for the patient's observations		
Requests sensible initial investigations to include Blood tests for FBC, CRP, LFTS, U&Es, Amylase and AXR / erect CXR or an ABG		
Differential Diagnosis – perforated peptic ulcer, pancreatitis, small bowel obstruction, mesenteric ischaemia, cholecystitis, gastritis, medical causes e.g. MI or LRTI		
Examiner's Global Mark	/5	
Actors Global Mark	/5	
Total Station Mark	/30	

Learning points:

Remember to adequately expose the patient. Examining around a patient gown can lead to missing pathology but the "Nipple to knee" approach is not appropriate for all patients – be guided by your findings.

Ensure you have a well-practiced slick method of examination. Start the examination of the abdomen by looking for peripheral stigmata of gastrointestinal disease.

Recognize that due to pain, your examination may need to be adapted so that you do not hurt the patient. Never forget that the genitalia should be examined as pain can radiate upwards and patients may feel shy in openly saying there is a problem.

45. Digital Rectal Examination

Student vignette

A 30-year-old man is attending the general surgical clinic with a history of persistent fresh bleeding from his back passage. You are the foundation year doctor in clinic with your registrar who asks you to perform a digital rectal examination on this patient. There will be a patient present in your station. You will be asked to initiate the consultation with the patient and explain the procedure to him.

You have 6 minutes after which you will then be asked by the examiner to list the features that you would examine during a digital rectal examination.

Actor Instructions:

You are a 30-year-old man named Simon attending a general surgery clinic appointment. Your GP has referred you as you have been having persistent bleeding from your back passage. The candidate has been asked to start a consultation with the aim of performing a digital rectal examination or examination of the back passage.

You will NOT be examined during this station, the candidate is required to discuss the examination with you only.

You should appear nervous during the consultation. The candidate should start by introducing themselves, explaining why they are here, explaining how the procedure will be carried out step by step, offer a chaperone and ask for your consent.

If the above aren't mentioned please ask the following of the candidate:
- Why do you need to feel my back passage when I have told you that I'm bleeding already?
- Do I have to be completely naked?
- Will it hurt?
- How long will it take?
- Tell the candidate that you feel uncomfortable and ask for reassurance
- If you are not offered, ask if you could have a member of the same sex present
- Can I refuse the examination?

Examiner Instructions:

The foundation year doctor has been asked to perform a digital rectal examination on this patient. There will be a patient present in the station. The candidate has been instructed to initiate the consultation with the patient and explain the procedure to him.

After 6 minutes stop the candidate and ask them to 'please summarise your findings, including a differential diagnosis and immediate management plan' for 2 minutes.

Please follow the mark sheet and grade appropriately.

Marksheet: DRE

Task:	Achieved	Not Achieved
Introduces self, washes hands and checks patient identity		
Puts patient at ease by asking patient how they are feeling or another type of generic question		
States aim of the consultation: to perform a digital rectal examination		
Explains to patient why this examination is necessary		
Offers the presence of a same sex chaperone		
Describes level of undress required: trousers and underwear pulled down to knees		
Reassures patient that a blanket will be provided for modesty		
Describes correct position for examination: laid flat on side, facing away and knees bent up to the chest		
Explains the examination with done with a single gloved finger and lubricating gel		
Warns the patient that they may be asked to gently squeeze around the finger or to describe if sensation is normal		
Encourages the patient to tell you to stop if they experience any pain or discomfort		
Explains that you will insert your finger anteriorly and gently sweep both clockwise and anti-clockwise		
Reassures the patient that the procedure should only last a few seconds		
Explains that the patient will be then be offered tissue and privacy to clean up		
Offers the patient the opportunity to ask questions		
Explicitly asks the patient for their consent		
Correctly states they would examine the external anus for skin changes and haemorrhoids		
States that they would assess anal tone		

States that they would feel for faeces, rectal masses and the prostate		
States that they would examine the glove for colour of faeces and blood		
Examiner's Global Mark	/5	
Actor / Helper's Global Mark	/5	
Total Station Mark	/30	

Learning Points

ALWAYS gain informed consent before undertaking any examination or procedure on a patient whether it be in your day to day practice or during an OSCE.

Potentially uncomfortable or intimate examinations are a good way to examine your communication skills in an OSCE. Remember to put the patient at ease, explain why the intimate examination is necessary and offer chaperones or alternative. Do not forget that patients have the right to refuse.

You will rarely be asked to actually perform intimate examinations, you will however be required to be able to describe the steps and what features you are examining. Therefore, do not discount intimate examinations during your revision.

46. Examination of Hernial Orifices

Student vignette

A 78-year-old man is referred to clinic with a large mass in his left groin. He does not describe any associated pain, nausea or vomiting. The patient is usually in good health, and is keen to be discharged from hospital.

You are the foundation year doctor on the surgical team and have been asked to examine the hernia, and present your findings to the examiner.

Actor Instructions:

You are Rafa, a 78-year-old male, having presented with a lump that appeared suddenly this morning following lifting heavy boxes into a van. You have presented because there is a large lump approximately the size of an orange that has appeared in your groin. It is tender to touch. You will be asked your identity and whether you consent to an examination of the lump to be performed. If the candidate fails to ask about a chaperone please prompt that you are not happy to proceed without one.

Examiner Instructions:

The foundation year doctor has been asked to perform an inguinal hernia examination.

After 6 minutes stop the candidate and ask them to 'please summarise your findings, including a differential diagnosis and immediate management plan' for 2 minutes.

Please follow the mark sheet and grade appropriately.

Marksheet: Hernial orifices

Task:	Achieved	Not Achieved
Introduces self, washes hands and checks patient identity		
Puts patient at ease by asking patient how they are feeling or another type of generic question		
States aim of the consultation: to perform an inguinal hernia examination		
Explains to patient why this examination is necessary		
Offers the presence of a same sex chaperone		
Describes level of undress required: trousers and underwear pulled down to knees		
Inspection of both inguinal regions, evaluating for size, induration and temperature check		
Observe cough impulse standing and lying		
Palpation of both inguinal regions		
Examination of the scrotum		
Feel for cough impulse on both sides		
Encourages the patient to tell you to stop if they experience any pain or discomfort		
Find deep inguinal ring		
Firmly press on lump and starting inferiorly lift the hernia up.		
Once reduced maintain pressure and assess cough impulse again		
Percussion of hernia		
Auscultation of hernia		
To complete examination- full abdominal and DRE required		
Summarize finding and investigations		
Able to differentiate between strangulated and incarcerated hernia		
Examiner's Global Mark	/5	
Actor / Helper's Global Mark	/5	
Total Station Mark	/30	

Learning points:

The difference between irreducible /incarceration/strangulation:

Irreducible – hernia that cannot be reduced to its original anatomical location.
Incarcerated – the contents of the hernia sac are stuck within the hernia sac
Strangulated –ischemia of the tissues contained within the hernia sac.

The mid-inguinal point is the halfway point between the anterior superior iliac spine and the pubic symphysis.

The anatomy borders for inguinal canal and femoral canal:

The inguinal canal is located above the medial half of the inguinal ligament. The inguinal ligament runs from the anterior superior iliac spine to the pubic tubercle. The inguinal canal has a deep inguinal ring located at the lateral aspect, and an external inguinal ring at the medial aspect.

The femoral canal is composed of:
Medial border – lacunar ligament
Lateral border – femoral vein
Anterior border – inguinal ligament
Posterior border – pectineal ligament, super pubic ramus and the pectineal muscle

The opening to the femoral canal is located at its superior border. This is known as the femoral ring.

47. Breast Examination

Student vignette

You are the foundation year doctor attending a Breast Surgical Clinic. Your consultant has asked you to perform a breast examination on Clarissa, a 49-year-old who has a lump in her right breast. Explain to the examiner what you are doing as you conduct your examination.

Please note that in the exam it is possible that you are given a model to perform the breast examination. But you will need to speak to the actor as though you are performing the examination on her.

Actor Instructions:

You are Clarissa a 49-year-old who has noticed a non-tender lump in your right breast. Do not offer any information to the candidate but you can respond to questions asking you whether you would like a chaperone and if you are in any pain, and be responsive to their instructions.

Examiner Instructions:

The foundation year doctor has been asked to perform a breast examination on a 49-year-old who has a lump in her right breast.

After 6 minutes stop the candidate and ask them to 'please summarise your findings, including a differential diagnosis and immediate management plan' for 2 minutes.

Please follow the mark sheet and grade appropriately.

Marksheet: Breast examination

Task:	Achieved	Not Achieved
Wash Hands, Introduction and Consent		
Requests a chaperone		
Expose & Position Patient		
Inspection: Asymmetry, Scars, Skin Changes, Nipple changes At Rest Patient tensing Pectoralis Muscles Patient's Hands behind Head axillae and inframmary folds		
Ask patient if she is in any pain before palpating the breasts.		
Palpation: Position- ipsilateral arm behind their head and tilt towards the contralateral side to flatten breast against chest wall Palpates breasts in a systematic manner Palpate the four quadrants, nipple areolar complex and the inframammary fold		
Feeling a Lump: Site, Size, Surface, Skin Changes Tenderness, Temperature Mobility and underlying attachment Fluctuant, compressible, pulsatile, Consistency		
Palpate B/L axillary tail of Spence and supraclavicular nodes		
Cover the patient, thank them and wash your hands		
Summary of Findings		
Initial investigations		
Management Plan		
Examiner's Global Mark	/5	
Actor / Helper's Global Mark	/5	
Total Station Mark	/30	

Learning Points

1. On inspection remember to look for any past signs of breast cancer such as mastectomy, scars, hair loss, radiation burns and lymphedema. As well as inspecting the back for latissimus dorsi flap reconstruction scars and the abdomen for TRAM flap reconstruction scars

2. Triple assessment for Breast Lump would be History & Examination (P1-5), Imaging – Mammography/USS (M1-5, U1-5) and Histology – Core Biopsy (B1-5)

3. Differential diagnosis for a breast lump: cancer, firboadenoma, cyst, abscess, fibrocystic change, lipoma, fat necrosis (20yrs – fibroadenoma, 40s – cyst, 70s – cancer).

48. Neck Lump and Thyroid examination

Student vignette

A 35-year-old woman has attended her GP practice complaining of anxiety and fatigue. You are the foundation year doctor on rotation and your GP supervisor asks you to do a full thyroid examination and present your findings.

You have 6 minutes after which you will be asked to summarise your findings and asked two questions about the examination.

Actor Instructions:

You are a 35-year-old woman named Susan, who attended her GP surgery complaining of anxiety and fatigue.
You have not noticed any skin or nail changes. You have not had any palpitations and not noticed any pain or swelling in the neck. You have not been feeling overly warm or cool recently and are dressed appropriately for the weather.

You should not feel any pain on examination. You should be asked to swallow sips of water and stick out your tongue by the candidate during the examination.

Examiner Instructions:

The foundation year doctor has been asked to do a full thyroid examination and present their findings. Please ensure a glass of water is available at the station.

After 6 minutes stop the candidate and ask them to 'please summarise your findings, including a differential diagnosis and immediate management plan' for 2 minutes.

Ask the candidate the following questions:

What clinical thyroid state is the patient in? Describe 2 differences on examination between a goitre and a thyroglossal cyst.

Please follow the mark sheet and grade appropriately.

Marksheet: Thyroid examination

Task:	Achieved	Not Achieved
Introduces self, washes hands and checks patient identity		
Explains examination, gains consent		
Asks patient to sit on a chair with neck and shoulders exposed		
Inspects hands, nails and skin		
Tests for fine tremor with a sheet of paper		
Looks for exophthalmos, lid lag and assesses eye movements		
Comments on clothing		
Inspects for signs of muscle wasting		
Looks for neck lump and scars		
Feels for radial pulse		
Feels for skin temperature		
Inspects for pre-tibial myxodema		
Palpates the thyroid and cervical nodes using a two handed technique and standing behind the patient asking them to tilt chin upwards.		
Asks patient to swallow water and observes/feels with one hand for movement of any neck lumps		
Asks patient to stick out tongue and observes/feels with one hand for movement of any neck lumps		
Auscultates for thyroid bruits		
Tests ankle reflexes		
Systematic presentation of findings		
Correctly identifies euthyroid state		
Identifies that: Both goitre and cyst move on swallowing but only cyst rises on tongue protrusion Cyst is soft whereas a goitre is hard +/- nodular		
Examiner's Global Mark	/5	
Actor / Helper's Global Mark	/5	
Total Station Mark	/30	

Learning Points

Practice presenting your examination findings in a systematic manner. Start by highlighting any obvious abnormality or state that this is a normal examination. Follow by summarising relevant positive findings and 2 to 3 significant negative findings. If it is a normal examination then state significant negatives and use opportunity to mention things you looked for but aren't necessarily obvious to the examiner. Conclude by offering a potential differential diagnosis or test that would help confirm diagnosis.

Know how to examine and describe a lump. There are many helpful mnemonics available. Most importantly always comment on site, size, shape, consistency and mobility. Top tip-soft is like your lips, firm is like the tip of your tongue and hard is like your nasal bridge.

When examining the cervical lymph nodes palpate using the pads of all four fingertips whilst standing behind the patient. Examine both sides at the same time. Walk your fingers along the pre-auricular, anterior cervical, posterior cervical, tonsilar, submandibular, submental and supraclavicular nodes.

49. Examination of Male Genitalia

Student vignette

You have been asked to see a 54-year-old male who is complaining of an abnormal lump and an uncomfortable dragging sensation in his left testis. You are the foundation doctor on the General Surgical Team and have been asked by your consultant to examine this patient. Please report your findings to the examiner.

Actor's Instructions

You are Thomas, a 54-year-old gentleman, who has presented complaining of an abnormal lump and dragging sensation in your left testis.

Do not offer any information to the candidate, however you can respond to questions asking whether you would like a chaperone and if you are in any pain.

Examiner's Instructions

The candidate has been asked to see a 54-year-old male who is complaining of an abnormal lump and an uncomfortable dragging sensation in his left testis.

There will be a patient present in the station. The candidate has been instructed to initiate the consultation with the patient and undertake an appropriate examination.

After 6 minutes stop the candidate and ask them to 'please summarise your findings, including a differential diagnosis and immediate management plan' for 2 minutes.

Please follow the mark sheet and grade appropriately.

Marksheet: Genital examination

Task	Achieved	Not Achieved
Introduces self, washes hands and checks patient identity		
Consent patients for examination		
Asks whether patient would like a chaperone		
Adequately exposes patient		
Performs general inspection of the patient notifying whether they are comfortable at rest or show signs of distress/compromise		
Observation of the groin Scrotal swellings Skin changes e.g. erythema, Surgical scars Discharge		
Palpation of testes Lump- size, shape, consistency (hard, firm, soft), Tenderness, Transillumination, painful/painless Palpates both sides Auscultates for bowel sounds		
Examines patient lying down		
Examines patient standing up		
Palpates associated structures- epididymis, ductus deferens.		
Examines glans penis Assesses phimosis, Lesions on penis		
Examines inguinal canal- Attempts to reduce lump if present Cough impulse to differentiate between direct and indirect hernia		
Palpates for enlarged inguinal and para-aortic lymph nodes.		
Examiner's Global Mark	/5	
Actor / Helper's Global Mark	/5	
Total Station Mark	/30	

Learning Points

Typically a varicocoele (dilatation of the pampiniform plexus veins) is described as feeling like "a bag of worms".

The gonadal vein on the right side drains directly in the IVC, however the vein on the left side drains into the left renal vein. Dilatation of the plexus on the left side may be indicative of a renal malignancy obstructing the left renal vein and causing back pressure .

Other differentials for testicular lumps include hydrocele (which would transilluminate), and an indirect inguinal hernia (cough impulse, bowel sounds).

50. ATLS Primary Survey

Student vignette

You are a foundation doctor working in the emergency department. A man is brought into resuscitation department, following a traumatic road traffic accident. You assess the patient along with an ED registrar, and an experienced ED nurse who will assist with tasks.

Your registrar requests you conduct the primary survey. Talk the examiner through how you would perform this and they will provide you with the clinical findings/observations/investigation results.

Actor Instructions:

You are a 25-year-old man, named Ben, who has just been knocked off your motorbike by a car turning out from a side road. You have significant pain in your neck and feel quite short of breath.

Follow the instructions of the doctor examining you.

Examiner's instructions:

The candidate has been asked to conduct a primary survey on a man brought into the resuscitation department, following a traumatic road traffic accident. The candidate has been instructed to talk you through the examination.

You must relay the below information to the candidate when it is appropriate. After 6 minutes, stop the candidate and ask them what further tests they would like to perform and for an immediate management plan.

	Observations	Clinical findings	Results
Airway		Airway is patent.	
C-spine		Patient has significant pain in the neck.	
Breathing	RR-22 Sats – 92%	Diminished air-entry on right. Percussion: more resonant on right. Asymmetrical chest wall movement (left > right). Trachea shifted to the left.	CXR – Right sided large pneumothorax.
Circulation	HR – 110 BP – 105/60	HS I+II+0 CRT 4 seconds. Cool peripheries. Patient slightly pale.	ECG – sinus tachycardia.
Disability	PEARL GCS: E4/V4/M6 Temp: 37	Blood glucose: 8	

The purpose of this task is to assess the following:

- An understanding of the ATLS assessment

Please follow the mark sheet and grade appropriately.

Marksheet: ATLS

Task:	Achieved	Not Achieved
Airway: Notes airway in patent		
C-spine: Elicits pain in patient's neck		
Immobilises patient's neck with blocks		
Breathing: Asks for RR and Saturations		
Chest wall movement/Percussion/Auscultation		
Trachea position		
Asks for CXR		
Suggests 15L oxygen non-rebreathe mask		
Circulations: Asks for HR and BP		
Capillary refill + pallor		
Heart sounds		
ECG		
Suggests large bore IV lines x2 and fluid bolus		
Recommends suitable blood test		
Disability: Pupils + GCS		
Blood sugar + temperature		
Mentions need for CT head + Chest/Abdomen/Pelvis		
Mentions need for full secondary survey for completion		
Mentions need to go back to A and continually reassess		
Suggests chest drain insertion for the pneumothorax		
Examiner's Global Mark	/5	
Actor / Helper's Global Mark	/5	
Total Station Mark	/30	

Learning points:

Remember in ATLS that assessment of the c-spine ALWAYS come in parallel with the airway.

It is important to be methodical and if you encounter an abnormality during your assessment to attempt an intervention before moving on. Even if there appears to be an obvious abnormality eg a deformed limb, stick to the A to E approach to avoid missing other more life threatening injuries

It is vital in these scenarios that you constantly go back and assess the patient again from the beginning to check for deterioration or success of intervention.

Peripheral Vascular Disease Examination

Student vignette

You have been asked to see a 72-year-old woman, who has presented to the vascular clinic complaining of pain in her calves on walking.

You are the foundation doctor on vascular team and have been asked by your consultant to conduct an examination of the peripheral vasculature. Please report your findings back to the examiner.

Actor's instructions

You are Bernadette, a 72-year-old woman, who has come to vascular clinic complaining of pain in your calves when walking. Do not offer any information to the candidate however you can respond to questions asking whether you would like a chaperone and if you are in any pain.

Examiner's Instructions

The candidate has been asked to see a 72-year-old woman who has presented to the vascular clinic complaining of pain in her calves on walking. There will be a patient present in the station.

The candidate has been instructed to conduct an examination of the peripheral vasculature and report their findings to you.

After 6 minutes stop the candidate and ask them to please summarise their findings.

Task	Achieved	Not Achieved
Introduces self, washes hands and checks patient identity		
Consents patient for examination		
Asks whether patient would like a chaperone present		
Adequately exposes the patient's lower limbs		
Performs a general observation of the patient noting whether they are comfortable at rest		
Observation of the lower limb: Scars from previous surgery Skin changes in colour / tissue loss. Venous eczema Presence of ulcers ensures to look all around the feet including heel		
Palpates temperature of both legs beginning distally		
Assesses capillary refill		
Performance of Buerger's tests if capillary refill is >2secs		
Performs palpation of pulses: Aorta Femoral Popliteal PT DT		
Checks for radiofemoral delay		
Auscultates for abdominal aortic bruits		
Correctly performs Doppler examination of the DP and PT pulse		
Correctly calculates the ABPI on both legs		
Examiner's Global Mark /5		
Actor / Helper's Global Mark /5		
Total Station Mark /30		

Learning Points

Presence of any varicose veins – often seen best with the patient standing up! Remember you should feel pulses on both sides and comment on their strength, comparing one side relative to the other.

Pulse Location:

Femoral - Mid inguinal point, halfway between the ASIS and the pubic symphysis

Popliteal - Deep in the popliteal fossa

Dorsalis Pedis - Between the head of the 1st and 2nd metatarsal

Posterior Tibial - Behind the medial malleolus

At the end, you should mention that you would perform a full cardiovascular system, examination the venous system in their legs and arrange an arterial duplex or angiogram.

21604276R00149

Printed in Great Britain
by Amazon